AROMATHERAPY,
MASSAGE AND
RELAXATION
IN CANCER CARE

of related interest

Essential Oils
A Handbook for Aromatherapy Practice
Second Edition
Jennifer Peace Rhind
ISBN 978 1 84819 089 4
eISBN 978 0 85701 072 8

The Spirit in Aromatherapy
Working with Intuition
Gill Farrer-Halls
ISBN 978 1 84819 209 6
eISBN 978 0 85701 159 6

Traditional Chinese Medicine Approaches to Cancer
Harmony in the Face of the Tiger
Henry McGrath
ISBN 978 1 84819 013 9
eISBN 978 0 85701 008 7

Getting Better at Getting People Better
Creating Successful Therapeutic Relationships
Noah Karrasch
ISBN 978 1 84819 239 3
eISBN 978 0 85701 186 2

Embroidered Cancer Comic
Sima Elizabeth Shefrin
ISBN 978 1 84819 289 8
eISBN 978 0 85701 237 1

Anni's Cancer Companion
An A–Z of Treatments, Therapies and Healing
Anni Matthews
ISBN 978 1 84819 067 2
eISBN 978 0 85701 044 5

AROMATHERAPY, MASSAGE AND RELAXATION IN CANCER CARE

An Integrative Resource for Practitioners

EDITED BY ANN CARTER
AND DR PETER A. MACKERETH

FOREWORDS BY ANNE CAWTHORN AND DEBORAH COSTELLO

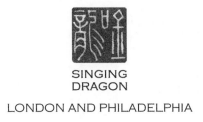

SINGING
DRAGON

LONDON AND PHILADELPHIA

Table 5.1 on pages 79–80 has been reprinted from Journal of Clinical Epidemiology, 58, 12, Boutron, I., Moher, D., Tugwell, P., Giraudeau, B. *et al.* 'A checklist to evaluate a report of non-pharmacological trial (CLEAR NPT) was developed using consensus.' 1233–1240, Copyright (2005), with permission from Elsevier.

First published in 2017
by Singing Dragon
an imprint of Jessica Kingsley Publishers
73 Collier Street
London N1 9BE, UK
and
400 Market Street, Suite 400
Philadelphia, PA 19106, USA

www.singingdragon.com

Library of Congress Cataloging in Publication Data
Names: Carter, Ann, editor. | Mackereth, Peter A., editor.
Title: Aromatherapy, massage, and relaxation in cancer care : an integrative resource for practitioners / edited by Ann Carter and Peter Mackereth ; forewords by Anne Cawthorn and Deborah Costello.
Description: London ; Philadelphia : Singing Dragon, 2017. | Includes bibliographical references and index.
Identifiers: LCCN 2016020121 | ISBN 9781848192812 (alk. paper)
Subjects: | MESH: Neoplasms--rehabilitation | Aromatherapy--methods | Relaxation Therapy--methods | Palliative Care--methods
Classification: LCC RC271.A62 | NLM QZ 200 | DDC 616.99406--dc23 LC record available at https://urldefense.proofpoint.com/v2/url?u=https-3A__lccn. loc.gov_2016020121&d=BQIFAg&c=euGZstcaTDllvimEN8b7jXrwqOf-v5A_CdpgnVfiiMM&r=VCKr2NBFNTs4O_kp07esGY2J-doQEb4zTq5sCaeXa-I&m=Xw3aFCQuStEcyKT-ZQNmSKS63rTeaClVY5IguCjnbKo&s=_wJSbsrLbPD4yN-TA8 EOXtwbwSGKjas9Pp4USqATvfU&e=

British Library Cataloguing in Publication Data
A CIP catalogue record for this book is available from the British Library

ISBN 978 1 84819 281 2
eISBN 978 0 85701 228 9

Printed and bound in Great Britain

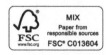

We dedicate this book to patients and carers who have contributed to our understanding of living with and recovering from cancer and its treatments. We acknowledge that learning is a two-way process with teachers (Ann and Peter) gaining invaluable insights and understanding from our students (therapists) who have attended our courses, workshops and conferences.

CONTENTS

FOREWORD

Anne Cawthorn

I was delighted to be asked to write a foreword to this book, not least because of my personal and professional journey with Peter and Ann as we have integrated complementary therapies into healthcare over the past 25 years. Although the therapies covered in this book are now adopted into the field of cancer and palliative care, this has not always been the case.

In the early days of introducing therapies I certainly recall sleepless nights, with many clinicians unconvinced as to the benefits of complementary therapies, and others worried about causing patients harm. Over the years much work has gone into 'changing hearts and minds'. This has taken the form of education, research and dissemination of good practice and even some receiving therapies to experience the benefits for themselves.

Education was one of the first obstacles to overcome, due to the lack of specialized courses in healthcare. Undaunted, the team developed therapy courses for those working in healthcare. The most important aspect of these courses has been to help therapists learn how to adapt and modify the therapies to safely meet the needs of patients living with cancer. Peter, Ann and the team have continued to further develop courses based on their innovative practice and have tirelessly disseminated this to others in the field of cancer care.

Through published service evaluations and research, they have provided much-needed evidence to underpin their clinical work. However, by far the greatest validation of the therapies has come from the patients and carers themselves. They have been instrumental in winning over clinicians as to the value of therapies in helping with the pain and symptoms relating to the disease and subsequent treatments, as well as improving resilience and wellbeing.

This book should prove an invaluable resource to any practitioner working in the field of cancer care who is interested in learning how research-based innovative therapies can be safely integrated into practice to enhance the care of patients and their carers.

Anne Cawthorn MBE, MSc, BSc, RN

FOREWORD

Deborah Costello

My name is Deborah Costello; I was 52 years old and came across a lump on my neck. I visited my GP and was referred to my local hospital to see what this was. The lump was removed under general anesthetic, and two weeks later I had the news that I needed to attend a cancer hospital for treatment. After a bone marrow biopsy and CT scan, the devastating news was given to me: I had chronic lymphocytic leukaemia.

After my first chemotherapy, I was given a large amount of take-home drugs, some of which I was dreadfully allergic to. I returned to the hospital and was introduced to Dr Jacqui Stringer (one of the contributors). She helped me make friends with the drugs that my body so very much needed.

Apart from my fabulous doctors and nurses, much-needed support came from the complementary therapy service, based on the Haematology Unit. As well as massage, I was introduced to aromasticks, where the scents trigger memories and allow the mind to rest and focus on alternatives to what treatment is being given, such as chemotherapy. The 'Stretchy Man' (a little rubber man with stretchy arms and legs) was used as a kind of stress ball. My 'Stretchy Man' became known as Peter, after Dr Peter A. Mackereth (co-editor of this book). It allowed me to picture his calm and soothing voice. I also experienced regular massages and creative imagery sessions while waiting for scans and tests.

In December 2010, I had the great news that I was in remission. Unfortunately in December 2011, my disease was back. I was told I needed a life-saving transplant. Again complementary therapies helped me enormously in dealing with this news. Hypnotherapy, acupuncture and massage all helped to keep my mind and body in good condition while waiting for a suitable donor. In November 2012, I received a bone marrow transplant. Complementary services were with me at every step of my recovery. This service was truly invaluable.

I was so pleased to hear that Ann and Peter had edited a new book about complementary therapies. As a service user I was also delighted to be asked if I could be involved through writing a foreword. I have met some of therapists involved in this book and I know they are committed to the use of complementary therapies in cancer care. I hope this book can help students and qualified therapists to develop their skills, so that more people affected by cancer can be assisted. The book will be an invaluable resource for anyone who wants to help improve the quality of life for people like me and my family.

Deborah Costello

ACKNOWLEDGEMENTS

The drive to develop this book came from our experience of delivering training, mentoring and supervising therapists and working with patients. Over the years we have, in our own inimitable way, contributed to challenging the myths around delivering complementary therapies to patients living with and recovering from cancer. These have included beliefs that massage spreads cancer and that the therapist may become contaminated with chemotherapy or radiotherapy from skin contact.

First, we would like to thank the therapists, patients, carers and volunteers who made the book possible. Additionally, we would like to thank the International Federation of Professional Aromatherapists, the Federation of Holistic Therapists and Denise Rankin-Box, Editor in Chief for the journal *Complementary Therapists in Clinical Practice*, for their support in publishing our articles, so helping us to shape our thinking and writing over many years.

We would like to thank Claire Wilson, Jane Evans and Alexandra Holmes from Jessica Kingsley Publishers for their interest in the book and for their support and advice.

Grateful thanks also to Stephen McGinn and Linda Orrett for their patience and expertise in information technology, having rescued us on several occasions.

Ann Carter and Dr Peter A. Mackereth

DISCLAIMER

Complementary therapy practices are constantly evolving in response to research, service evaluations, needs of patients (and carers) and concurrent development in medical practice. It is the responsibility of the therapist to maintain professional development and to work within the policies and practices in the context of his/her own clinical and private practice. The contributors and publisher are not responsible for any harm or damage to a person, no matter how caused, as a result of information shared in this book.

INTRODUCTION AND AN OVERVIEW OF THE BOOK

The numbers of people being diagnosed and living with the consequences of cancer and its treatments are growing. Complementary therapy provision is expanding in public and private services, with the need to safely adapt therapeutic skills built on evidence-based knowledge to meet the challenges of clinical and private practice. People living with and recovering from cancer treatment drive the development of quality care, with therapists having accountability and responsibility to hone their practice to be effective and compassionate. Empathic responses include an appreciation of the physical, emotional and spiritual complexities of a cancer diagnosis and its consequences. No cancer journey is the same for every individual, their families and friends; we need to be mindful to their uniqueness, be in the moment and skilfully adapt our interventions.

Within this book we have brought together skilled and experienced contributors to link theory with practice, with the purpose of enriching the quality of complementary care offered in cancer services. Patient choices and therapist options are key elements that can come together like the pieces of a jigsaw puzzle to make a therapeutic interaction a meaningful, holistic experience. Patients, carers, multidisciplinary colleagues and therapists, working together and sharing experiences, can effect change in terms of service provision, understanding and the valuing of complementary therapies. Contributors to this book are involved in a variety of complementary therapy and cancer care settings, sharing a plethora of approaches, techniques and adaptions to equip novice and experienced practitioners in expanding their therapeutic toolbox.

In seeking and selecting this book for your development and studies, we recognize that you are engaged in a process of exploration and discovery. We hope that within these pages the content will assist you in becoming even more creative in maximizing your therapeutic skills. We recognize that this book is part of a worldwide movement to acquire the necessary evidence and experience to enable greater interaction and appreciation of complementary therapy approaches to cancer care.

The book is divided into two parts; the first is concerned with the principles that underpin clinical practice and the context of our work. The second is concerned with innovative and practical applications of the three complementary therapies, aromatherapy, massage and relaxation. Where possible, the content in the chapters has been cross-referenced to reinforce and demonstrate the interweaving of practice. We have included composite case histories, which help to illustrate the principles discussed. All chapters begin with key words and a short introduction.

Part 1 begins with the chapter Cancer and Its Treatments, which details the causes and treatments of cancer from a clinical perspective. Chapters 2 and 3 focus on two key 'players' in the forming of a therapeutic relationship: the patient and the complementary therapist. Much of the content of the book also applies to carers, so where we have put 'patient' most of the principles and suggestions could be applicable to both. Chapter 2, The Resilient Patient, explores the concept of resilience, its relevance to patients with cancer and the therapist's role in helping patients to access resources. Chapter 3 focuses on the role of the therapist and how therapists can stay resourceful when faced with the challenges of working in clinical settings. Chapter 4 is concerned with documentation. Bearing in mind the legal requirements for well-documented notes, this chapter explains the values of policies and standard operating procedures and how they can be useful to the therapist. A method of auditing is suggested to assess how effective the documentation is when it is in use. In Chapter 5, we cover the issues involved in research and interpreting research for therapists, and provide examples of research summaries that relate to the three therapies featured in the book. It is not always possible or appropriate for therapists to carry out formal research. However, monitoring and evaluating an existing or a new service can provide valuable information, not only for review but also in seeking longer-term funding and acceptance. Chapter 6 is a case study reviewing data of a palliative care therapy service seeking to become embedded within an acute cancer setting.

The content of Part 1 underpins our work as complementary therapists and offers a foundation to support the practical applications discussed in Part 2 of this book.

The first three chapters in Part 2 are concerned with exploring the role of essential oils in clinical and supportive care settings. The first chapter (Chapter 7), Aromatherapy: The SYMPTOM Model, has been designed to help therapists work effectively in cancer care settings as part of the multidisciplinary team, integrating complementary therapies within clinical care. In recent times, aromasticks have become increasingly popular and Chapter 8 covers a variety of ways of using this very useful tool, particularly when combined with different approaches to guided imagery. Chapter 9 discusses the problems of malodour with reference to the potential use of essential oils to meet some of the challenges faced by patients, families, visitors and staff.

The next two chapters (Chapters 10 and 11) explore progressive muscle relaxation (PMR) and guided imagery (GI) in some depth. The chapter on PMR explores the approach to helping patients learn the technique, together with some suggestions about managing groups effectively. The focus is a 'drop-in' model, where the group membership can change each time it is held. In the chapter on guided imagery, we discuss the use of scripts and how to work with patients in a person-centred way. Chapter 12 is focused on The HEARTS[1] Process and details some 'hands-on' approaches, combining ways of using imagery, working over clothing and integrating the senses. Chapter 13 covers techniques which can be used to help patients who have difficulty in breathing; these can be taught to build respiratory resilience and ease breathing during acute situations. Chapter 14 focuses on the needs of carers and the potential for the use of the massage chair. The final chapter in the book raises some of the spiritual and ethical dilemmas surrounding massage (and other therapies) at the end of life, making recommendations for working helpfully at this challenging time.

---

1   'Hands-on, Empathy, Aromas, Textures and Sound'

Part 1

Part 1

UNDERLYING PRINCIPLES OF CLINICAL PRACTICE

Chapter 1

CANCER AND ITS TREATMENTS

Timothy Jackson

KEY WORDS
cancer, causes, staging, chemotherapy,
radiotherapy, surgery, palliative care

INTRODUCTION

This chapter provides an introduction to cancer care, possible causes, and an overview of symptoms, investigations and treatment modalities. More people are living with cancer and/or recovery from treatment. As a consequence, there is a need to adjust to longer-term side-effects and ongoing monitoring for disease recurrence or progression. We recommend that therapists maintain and develop their knowledge, and work to be part of a patient-centred multidisciplinary team.

THE NATURE OF CANCER

Cancer covers over 200 different diseases sharing common characteristics, including the uncontrolled division of cells, which can invade other adjacent tissues and/or migrate to distant sites (*metastasis*) in the body (Hirsch, Kett and Trefil 2002). Cells in different parts of the body may look and work differently but all reproduce themselves in an orderly and controlled manner. New cells can develop to form a tumour when division processes malfunction; a tumour can either be benign (*it does not spread*) or malignant (*it can spread or metastasize*). Cancers can be broadly grouped into different types, depending on which tissues they come from; they are often referred to as solid tumours or liquid cancers. Examples of solid tumours include breast and lung cancer; examples of liquid tumours are leukaemias (blood cancers) or myeloma (cancer of the white cells). Another classification is to refer to groups of cancers as 'common' or 'rare' cancers, depending on their incidence per head of population. These cancers can occur at any age, although there is a higher incidence in some age groups, such as children and young people with, for example, the rare soft tissue or bone sarcoma. Some of the most common solid cancers include breast, lung, colorectal, gynaecological and prostate.

CAUSES AND PROGNOSIS

The etiology of cancer is not fully understood, but it is thought to be caused by a combination of factors. Acknowledged factors include substances, such as the use of tobacco (including passive smoking), alcohol and drugs, exposure to radiation (ionizing and solar), genetic predisposition, contact with viruses and/or parasites, and immunological deficiencies. Additionally, dietary factors, obesity, food contaminants, occupational hazards and environmental pollution have also been implicated (Eriksen, Mackay and Ross 2012; Parkin, Boyd and Walker 2011; Secretan *et al.* 2009).

DIAGNOSIS

The early detection of cancer is very important to ensure early treatment and improved survival. Some of the signs and symptoms that require investigation include:

- a new or unusual lump anywhere on the body
- a mole which changes in shape, size or colour
- a sore that will not heal (including in the mouth)
- a persistent problem, such as persistent coughing or hoarseness
- a change in bowel or urinary habits
- any abnormal bleeding, such as blood in the stool or urine
- unexplained weight loss.

(based on Europe Against Cancer 1995)

After the initial diagnosis, the term 'staging' is used to describe whether the cancer is localized or if there is lymph nodal involvement and/or metastatic spread. When patients are diagnosed, they are 'staged' with levels 1–4. Stage 1 indicates that the tumour is isolated with no local spread. If there is some local spread to the lymphatic nodes, this is referred to as stage 2. Stage 3 is where there is both local spread and also secondary cancers or metastases in nearby organs. Stage 4 is where there is wide spread of the cancer cells to the lymphatic system in the chest and abdomen, with a number of metastases across several major organs (Souhami and Tobias 2005). The process of staging can be a useful prognostic guide. Stages 1 and 2 often present with a good (or better outcome) and prognosis than stages 3 or 4; it follows that awareness and detection are key to improved survival. However, for a number of patients, the initial diagnosis is as a consequence of an emergency presentation such as bowel obstruction for colorectal cancers, epileptic seizure for a brain tumour, or widespread bruising when presenting with a leukaemia.

Variables such as sex or age can also be important to the progress of certain cancers. For example, children, teenagers and young adults generally present with rarer and more aggressive cancers, which are responsive to curative high-dose therapies. In older people, some cancers may be controlled or held in remission with ongoing treatment modalities. For example, some forms of prostate cancer can be managed by endocrine treatments, helping to contain disease progression and extend life (DeSantis *et al.* 2014). Prognosis is dependent on a number of factors, such as stage at presentation, age, gender, genetic or chromosomal abnormalities and co-morbidities. Therefore, cancer treatment is now becoming more tailored to the individual with the introduction of personalized medicine.

DIAGNOSTICS

Diagnosis of cancer can be achieved in several ways, for example following a full physical examination by an experienced clinician or from blood tests, such as a full blood count for leukaemia. Tests include radiological examinations (x-rays and mammography) and biopsy of the tumour using endoscopy or surgery. More sophisticated diagnostic technologies such as computerized tomography, magnetic resonance imaging (MRI) and positron emissions tomography (PET scan) are now readily available and routine. Over the last decade, the development of personalized cancer care and the investment in treatment have improved. Contributing factors have been an improvement in accurate and more precise tissue typing, together with developments in skills and techniques in histopathology and radiology, new systemic anti-cancer technologies, surgical and anaesthetic techniques.

AN OVERVIEW OF CANCER TREATMENT

Surgery

First, some surgery can be diagnostic and includes biopsies and endoscopies. Second, definitive surgery aims to remove as much of the tumour as possible, along with a clear margin of healthy tissue that surrounds it, the purpose being to achieve a cure. Nearby lymph nodes are often removed to check for any spread of the cancer. Surgical treatments can be so extensive that removal of a tumour may require amputation of a limb or pelvic clearance of a number of organs. Debulking of the tumour is sometimes necessary to remove as much of the tumour as possible prior to chemotherapy or radiotherapy treatments. This has enormous implications for recovery, rehabilitation and body image. Palliative surgery is sometimes carried out to relieve symptoms of advanced cancer. It may also be necessary to insert medical devices, such as feeding tubes and stents (a rigid tube inserted to maintain an opening in a body canal, such as the oesophagus). These interventions can help to improve a patient's quality of life for as long as possible. The indications for surgery can also be prophylactic where a person has an increased genetic risk, for example where a woman has the breast cancer gene. Additionally, some patients may also require reconstructive surgery, for example, following a mastectomy. Surgical techniques and enhanced recovery pathways are improving yearly, enabling patients with, for example, breast cancer, to have surgery as a day case. Where patients have common cancers that do not require complex surgery, the operation is often performed in local district general-style hospitals. For patients with complex, rare or anatomically difficult tumours, these are often treated in specialist centres. Access to other co-dependent services may be essential; these include neurosurgery, thoracic surgery and/or liver transplant expertise for patients presenting with a hepato-biliary cancer or pancreatic cancer.

Systemic anti-cancer therapy

Systemic anti-cancer therapy is the collective heading given to drugs or biological therapies that either kill cancer cells or interfere in cell production by preventing cancer cell duplication. Both systemic anti-cancer therapies and radiotherapy treatments involve the exploitation of the biological characteristics of cancer cells to make them susceptible to drug therapy. Both radiotherapy and chemotherapy exert their initial effects more effectively in cancer cells; normal cells have intact genetic machinery which offers protection (Casciato and Territo 2012, first published 1995). Cytotoxic chemotherapy or 'chemo' is the commonly used term given to the drugs that kill cancer cells. Cytotoxic chemotherapy prevents the cancerous cells from developing and multiplying. Different chemotherapies are administered to prevent cell division and replication during the different stages of cell division. The aim is to maximize cell kill, commonly known as the 'cell kill hypothesis', by giving therapy doses over a number of days or weeks, therefore killing cancer cells and preventing further regrowth – see Figure 1.1.

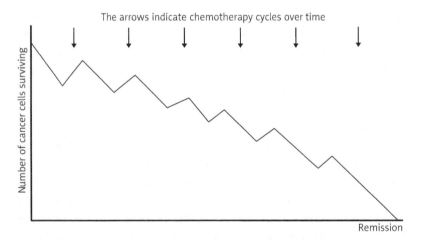

Figure 1.1: Cancer cell kill hypothesis with chemotherapy
(adapted from Souhami and Tobias 2005; Casciato and Territo 2012, first published 2000)

Cycles of different types of chemotherapy affecting different phases of cell division are given to maximize cell kill and minimize unwanted side-effects. The treatment is given at intervals to allow recovery and at the same time prevent or minimize tumour growth. The aim of treatment is to completely destroy the tumour over a period of time. Side-effects are divided into short, medium and long term; their longevity is dependent on the type and dosage of chemotherapy. Monitoring of prompt recognition for signs and symptoms of side-effects and immediate treatment and care is paramount in oncology patients. Details of the side-effects of these treatments are given below. While some chemotherapy can be given orally, or via a tunnelled intravenous cannula, many patients require a peripheral cannula – see Figure 1.2.

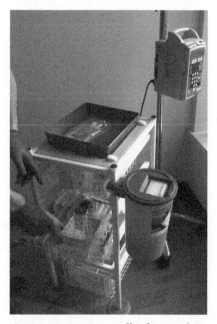

Figure 1.2: Preparing a trolley for cannulation

For some patients, repeated needling can be distressing and may require interventions to prevent panic and phobic responses (Mackereth and Tomlinson 2014). Chemotherapy-related fatigue as a persisting side-effect is increasingly being recognized by health professionals. This condition can severely limit both the ability to return to work and maintain activities of daily living. Fatigue can also compromise mood, social and family life, and affect sexual functioning and memory (Mackereth *et al.* 2015).

Systemic anti-cancer therapy/cytotoxic chemotherapy side-effects include:

- Immediate: anaphylaxis, nausea, vomiting, chemical cystitis, flushing.

- Short and medium term: diarrhea, constipation, dry mouth, loss of appetite, anorexia, peripheral neuropathy, menopause, loss of sleep, fatigue, altered body image.

- Long term: hair loss, altered body image, loss of function, infertility, anaemia, neutropenia (predisposition to infect-ion), thrombocytopenia (predisposition to bruising and/ or hemorrhage), pancytopenia (which means anemia, thrombocytopenia and neutrophenia), insomnolance, cardiac and renal, hepatic impairment, premature menopause, fatigue, psychological and sociological effects.

- Rare side-effects: kidney damage, liver damage, heart failure including cardiac-conduction-electrical and cardio myopathy, peripheral neuropathy (tingling in the hands and feet), damage to the bladder lining, tinnitus (ringing in the ears).

(based on Dougherty and Bailey 2001)

Opportunist infections, which can be present in 'healthy' people with functioning immune systems, can be life-threatening for the neutropenic (low white cells) patient. Opportunistic infections include bacteria, viruses, such as herpes zoster (shingles) or fungal infections, such as aspergillus. Infection may be detected through physical examination of the skin, mouth, and intravenous sites or through microbiological examination. It can be difficult to assess in patients with low white blood cells as there may be no signs of inflammation. If a patient with neutropenia has a systemic infection, there may only be evidence of a raised temperature. A temperature of 38°C or above requires immediate treatment with intravenous powerful antibiotics. If left untreated, septic shock may develop and death may occur within a few hours or days. It is important to provide information to enable patients (and carers) to understand their disease and its treatment, so that they can make choices about their care. The side-effects caused by the chemotherapy may require additional supportive care and/or further medication.

Examples of conventional management for side-effects of chemotherapy include:

- antiemetics for nausea and vomiting

- analgesia for pain, plus other drugs, known as co-analgesics, for example steroids, that can help to reduce swelling and inflammation, which in turn reduces pain

- intravenous fluids for dehydration (for example, due to diarrhea or nausea and vomiting), plus additional electrolytes such as minerals, for example potassium or calcium for electrolyte disturbance

- aperients or laxatives for constipation

- blood product transfusion such as packed red cells for anaemia or platelets to prevent or stop bleeding

- antibiotics, antiviral drugs or antifungal drug therapy for infections.

(based on Edwards 2003)

Hormones

Hormone therapy can play a part in the management of cancer and its symptoms. It can be given to treat and/or control certain cancers, such as breast or prostate cancer. The therapy works by leading to a fall in certain hormones that would otherwise increase tumour size and activity. Common side-effects, for example in hormone therapy for prostate cancer, include: hot flushes, weight gain, erectile dysfunction and emotional changes (Banks 2004).

Corticosteroids

Corticosteroids can be used where tumours have been complicated by local inflammation and edema. These conditions can obstruct nerve pathways and cause pain and/or alteration in sensation. Corticosteroids can also be used for chemotherapy-induced nausea, with or without an antiemetic (Casciato and Territo 2012). Steroids, such as synthetic glucocorticoids, have potent anti-inflammatory action, which can reduce edema around the tumour. They are commonly used to relieve symptoms or immediately prior to the start of emergency radiotherapy or surgery for metastatic spinal cord compression. Additionally, they can also be used for cerebral edema caused by primary or secondary brain tumours (Souhami and Tobias 2005). Prolonged use of steroids suppresses the development of white blood cells in the bone marrow, leading to infection. However, steroids can be beneficial as an essential treatment adjuvant (an agent which modifies the effects of other agents) in patients presenting with a leukemia.

Stratified cancer drug treatment

Technologies for cancer treatment are improving; there are now a number of licensed medicines which have been designed to target specific genetic mutations or other abnormalities in a patient's cancer. These targeted medicines can improve outcomes for certain patient groups, providing greater progression-free or overall survival and avoidance of undesirable side-effects for those patients for whom these treatments will not work. Patients can experience many months or years of extra survival plus a much better quality of life depending on the type of cancer and specific medicine.

Radiotherapy

Radiotherapy is an intervention that uses ionizing radiation, the goal being to destroy or inactivate cancer cells, while preserving the integrity of adjacent healthy tissues. A machine called a linear accelerator, which looks like a large x-ray machine, delivers radiotherapy. The treatment is measured in units called fractions, which usually takes several minutes to complete. Treatment planning takes into account a number of factors, including the cancer site(s), sensitivity to radiotherapy, and staging of the cancer. The daily dose can be distributed over a time span which can run into weeks (Faithfull 2001). Each time, patients must be placed in the exact same position for the treatment, with the area(s) marked. Immobilization and positioning devices, such as masks, casts and arm boards, are sometimes necessary to ensure stabilization and accuracy of targeted delivery (see Figure 1.3). For patients these treatments, associated scans and immobilization devices can trigger feelings of anxiety, distress and claustrophobia (Mackereth *et al.* 2012).

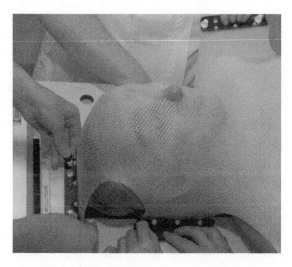

*Figure 1.3: An immobilization mask used in head
and neck radiotherapy treatments*

Recent advances in radiotherapy using cutting-edge imaging and computing technology have helped to target radiation doses more precisely. As a result, these procedures enable better outcomes, with improved quality of life for patients. Precision radiotherapy (or stereotactic radiotherapy) ensures that radiotherapy is precisely delivered to the tumour in areas that have been previously difficult to treat. Intraoperative radiotherapy is administered directly to the tumour site following removal of the tumour while the patient is on the operating table. This avoids the challenge of daily courses of radiotherapy over several weeks, which is extremely demanding for patients and costly for the health economy. This method releases resources and increases capacity for other patients requiring radiotherapy. Brachytherapy involves radioactive sources being positioned within a body cavity, or tissue, close to the tumour. The tumour receives a higher and more direct dose, with less radiation affecting the surrounding healthy tissue. These sealed sources can be left in position for a few minutes or a few hours. This treatment can be used for certain cancers such as tongue, breast, uterine and cervical cancers (Devlin 2007). Unsealed source therapy (radioactive liquids) is given as an injection or a drink, which targets a particular type of tissue, for example radioactive iodine for thyroid cancer, radioactive strontium for prostate cancer which has spread to the bones, and radioactive phosphorous for certain malignant blood disorders. Cesium 125 is a radioactive element which is put into an applicator and then inserted into the vagina and cervix. This is known as cesium insertion, with patients having this procedure under a general anaesthetic. Some patients will have cesium insertion and be connected to a selectron machine. This machine loads the radioactive material into the applicator once the patient has returned from theatre. Patients are nursed in isolation, following strict radiation protection guidelines and policies. Treatment lasts for 12–48 hours and the patient is observed on close-circuit television. Opening the door to the room switches off the machine, so any undue interruptions will prolong the length of time in isolation, which may be very distressing for the patient. An example of a new form of therapy is proton beam, which is in its infancy in the UK; unlike conventional radiotherapy, the beam of protons stops once it 'hits' the cancerous cells (Gerweck and Paganetti 2008).

Side-effects of radiotherapy

Patients receiving radiotherapy may experience two common side-effects: skin reactions and fatigue. Skin reactions are site-specific, and the skin in the treatment field may become reddened and sore. Patients are advised to wear loose clothing and use non-scented toiletries. If the skin reaction is severe, treatment may have to be temporarily suspended. Fatigue is recognized as a common occurrence with radiotherapy. It usually begins during treatment and can persist for days and even weeks. The causes of fatigue are not fully understood; some contributing factors include the accumulation of metabolites, cell destruction and the need for resources for tissue repair (Ahlberg, Ekman and Gaston-Johansson 2005; Molassiotis and Chan 2004). Long-term side-effects can occur and are anatomically related to the area irradiated. For example, in head and neck radiation, side-effects can include altered taste sensation, and long-term dryness of the mouth where the salivary glands have been irradiated. In breast cancer, lymphoedema may occur where lymph nodes have received radiotherapy, and in colon cancer, constipation or loose stools/diarrhea may occur as a result of radiation.

Transplants

For patients with a leukaemia or lymphoma-type cancer, treatment can also include 'a transplant' from either an allogeneic donor (who may be a relative or unrelated) or using tissues from themselves (an autologous donor). This process can be carried out once the patient is in remission and the aim is to ensure cure or long-term survival. Several years ago, the donor or patient's bone marrow was harvested. This older technology is being replaced by technology called aphaeresis, where the required cells are taken from the patient's blood and the remainder is returned to the circulation.

CANCER TREATMENT SURVEILLANCE AND ACUTE ONCOLOGY SERVICES

As highlighted in the above sections, treatment, and sometimes the cancer, can cause unpleasant or life-threatening side-effects. To improve the care, treatment, experience and outcomes for patients suffering from these side-effects, a number of services and strategies have been developed over the last few years.

The role of supportive and palliative care

Improving Supportive and Palliative Care for Adults with Cancer (NICE Guidance 2004) highlights key supportive and palliative care interventions that build a bundle of care (see Box 1.1). The care starts at diagnosis and concludes when the person completes living with and beyond the cancer programme of care, before being finally discharged. This approach recognizes that for some cancer patients, living with and beyond cancer may still require long-term support and care. Their ongoing needs may be either as a consequence of their treatment, or ongoing progressive disease or co-morbidity. This is a particular challenge in cancer, with the myriad problems a diagnosis can bring and the increasing number of co-morbidities patients have to cope with. For example, a patient with a history of heavy smoking may have lung cancer and pre-existing chronic obstructive pulmonary disease (COPD). He/she may require cancer treatment, plus support to stop smoking and manage breathlessness, fatigue and a cough.

Box 1.1: Supportive and palliative care interventions

- self-help and support
- information-giving
- psychological support
- symptom control
- social support
- rehabilitation including management of lymphoedema
- complementary therapies
- spiritual support
- palliative care
- end-of-life and bereavement care.

(NICE 2004)

Rehabilitation and survivorship

Rehabilitation aims to restore a person's roles and functions as far as possible, and to help him/her to adjust to limitations where required. These roles and functions may be relevant to any context, including family, society or returning to work. Effective rehabilitation is vital in minimizing consequences of treatment and improving quality of life for someone with cancer. Preventative rehabilitation can be delivered before and during cancer treatment; it also has the potential to reduce the future clinical and non-clinical needs of a person with cancer. This could, in turn, reduce the cost to the health and social care system associated with later stage and more serious interventions. Better support for people after treatment can deliver significant benefits in terms of improved quality of life. It can also encourage healthier lifestyles that are more likely to prevent recurrence or acute presentations back to the health service with late consequences of treatment. For example, there is strong evidence that patients who are encouraged to undertake a programme of physical activity post-treatment suffer from reduced levels of fatigue and have overall higher quality of life, across a range of cancer types. Importantly, being smoking-free during and beyond cancer treatment can reduce the risks of recurrence, new disease(s) and exacerbating longer-term side-effects across many cancers (Baile 2008; Sarna, Grannis and Coscarelli 2007). Health professionals are recognizing that patients (and carers) can experience a care 'void' from diminishing acute cancer support/monitoring. This is compounded by post-traumatic stress from the initial diagnosis/treatment experience, fear of, or anxious monitoring for, recurrence and the burden of longer-term side-effects (Ganz 2007).

Palliative care

Palliative care has been defined as 'the active holistic care of patients with advanced, progressive illness' (NICE 2004, p.20). Its aim is to maximize quality of life for patients and carers and it includes the management of symptoms alongside providing other forms of support. Approaches may offer support for physical symptoms such as pain, as well as helping with symptoms of an emotional, psychological or spiritual nature. Often, 'palliative care' is a term used where disease is advanced. This may be a cause of concern to some patients and their families; palliation is often associated with advanced disease and for patients who are dying. Increasingly, however, palliative care teams are supporting patients at an earlier stage in their cancer pathway. Pennell and Corner (2001, p.518) state that 'palliative care is argued as useful throughout the cancer journey'. The aims of palliative care include:

- Provide relief from pain and other distressing symptoms.

- Integrate the psychological and spiritual aspects of patient care.

- Offer a support system to help patients to live as actively as possible until death.

- Help the family to cope during the patient's illness and in their own bereavement.

- To be applied early in the course of illness in conjunction with other therapies intended to prolong life (such as chemotherapy or radiation therapy), including investigations to better understand and manage distressing clinical side-effects.

(NICE 2004, p.20)

SUMMARY

Cancer care, treatment and outcomes for people affected by cancer have improved over the last 15 years. However, the increased incidence and earlier diagnosis of cancer means that there is still more to do in developing new technologies for treating patients. Therapists can play an important role in supporting patients (and carers) throughout and beyond their cancer treatment. Additionally, therapists can have a role in promoting early diagnosis and treatment by encouraging patients with symptoms or concerns to attend for medical screening and review. Importantly, we can all encourage and support patients, carers (and colleagues) to make lifestyle changes to improve health and wellbeing and reduce risks of disease and/or recurrence.

REFERENCES

Ahlberg, K., Ekman, T., Gaston-Johansson, F. (2005) 'The experience of fatigue, other symptoms and global quality of life during radiotherapy for uterine cancer.' *International Journal of Nursing Studies 42,* 4, 377–386.

Baile, W.F. (2008) 'Alcohol and nicotine dependency in patients with head and neck cancer.' *Journal of Supportive Oncology 6,* 165–166.

Banks, I. (2004) *The Cancer Manual.* England: Haynes Publishing.

Casciato, D. and Territo, M.C. (2012) *Manual of Clinical Oncology,* Seventh Edition. Philadelphia: Lippincott, William and Wilkins.

Corner, J. and Bailey, C. (2001) *Cancer Nursing: Care in Context.* Oxford: Blackwell Science Ltd.

Department of Health (2007) *Cancer Reform Strategy.* London: DoH.

Department of Health (2011) *Improving Outcomes: A Strategy for Cancer.* London: DoH.

Department of Health (2010) *National Cancer Survivorship Initiative Vision Document.* London: DoH.

DeSantis, C.E., Lin, C.C., Mariotto, A.B., Siegal. R.L. *et al.* (2014) 'Cancer treatment and survivorship statistics 2014'. *A Cancer Journal for Clinicians 64,* 4, 252–271.

Devlin, P.M. (2007) *Brachytherapy: Applications and Techniques.* Philadelphia: Lippincott Williams and Wilkins.

Dougherty, L. and Bailey, C. (2001) 'Chemotherapy' In J. Corner and C. Bailey (eds) *Cancer Nursing: Care in Context.* Oxford: Blackwell Science Ltd.

Edwards, S.J. (2003) 'Prevention and treatment of adverse effects related to chemotherapy for recurrent ovarian cancer.' *Seminars in Oncology Nursing. 19,* 3, Suppl. 1:19–39.

Eriksen, M., Mackay, J., Ross, H. (2012) *The Tobacco Atlas.* Atlanta: American Cancer Society.

Europe Against Cancer (1995) *European 10-Point Code.* London: Working Party on European Code.

Faithfull, S. (2001) 'Radiotherapy.' In J. Corner and C. Bailey (eds) *Cancer Nursing: Care in Context.* Oxford: Blackwell Science Ltd.

Ganz, P.A. (2007) 'Cancer Survivors: A Physician's Perspective.' In P. A. Ganz (ed.) *Cancer Survivorship: Today and Tomorrow.* New York: Springer.

Gerweck, L. and Paganetti, H. (2008) 'Radiobiology of Charged Particles.' In T.F. Delaney and H.M. Kooy (eds) *Proton and Charged Particle Radiotherapy.* Philadelphia, PA: Lippincott Williams and Wilkins.

Hirsch, E.D. Jr., Kett, J.F., Trefil, J. (eds) (2002) *The New Dictionary of Cultural Literacy.* Boston, MA: Houghton Mifflin Company.

Mackereth, P. and Tomlinson, L. (2014) 'Procedure-related anxiety and needle phobia: rapid techniques to calm.' *Nursing in Practice 80,* 55–57.

Mackereth, P., Bardy, J., Finnegan-John, J., Farrell, C., Molassiotis, A. (2015) 'Legitimising Fatigue After Breast Cancer Treatment: The 'Coping with Fatigue' Booklet. *British Journal of Nursing 24,* 4, S4–12.

Mackereth, P., Tomlinson, L., Maycock, P., Donald, G. *et al.* (2012) 'Calming panic states in the mould room and beyond: a pilot complementary therapy head and neck service.' *Journal of Radiotherapy in Practice 11,* 2, 83–91.

Molassiotis, A. and Chan, C.W.H. (2004) 'Fatigue patterns in Chinese patients receiving radiotherapy.' *European Journal of Oncology Nursing 8,* 4, 334–340.

National Institute for Clinical Excellence (2004) *Improving supportive and palliative care for adults with cancer: the manual.* London: National Institute for Clinical Excellence.

Parkin, D.M., Boyd, L., Walker, L.C. (2011) 'The fraction of cancer attributable to lifestyle and environmental factors in the UK in 2010.' *British Journal of Cancer 105,* Suppl: S77–81.

Pennell, M. and Corner, J. (2001) 'Palliative Care and Cancer.' In J. Corner and C. Bailey (eds) *Cancer Nursing: Care in Context.* Oxford: Blackwell Science Ltd.

Sarna, L., Grannis, Jr, F.W., Coscarelli, A. (2007) 'Physical and Psychological Issues in Lung Cancer Survivors.' In P. A. Ganz (ed.) *Cancer Survivorship: Today and Tomorrow.* New York: Springer.

Secretan, B., Straif, K., Baan, R. Grosse, Y. *et al.* (2009) 'A review of human carcinogens – Part E: tobacco, areca nut, alcohol smoke, and salted fish.' *The Lancet Onocology 10,* 11, 1033–1034.

Souhami, R. and Tobias, J. (2005) *Cancer and its Management.* Oxford: Blackwell Science.

Chapter 2

THE RESILIENT PATIENT
Lynne Tomlinson

KEY WORDS
resilience, patients, allies, resources, self-reflective questions, choice

INTRODUCTION

The concept of resilience provides therapists with a rich opportunity to nurture a patient's self-care practices, within the shelter of a therapeutic relationship and environment. This chapter considers helpful definitions of resilience and resilience processes emerging from the research. It also highlights the dynamic and evolving nature of the concept of resilience. Examples of case histories are used to demonstrate supportive interventions during moments of patient and carer vulnerabilities and transitions. Finally, self-reflective questions are offered to help you identify what exemplifies resilience for yourself, and how to integrate resilience-building into your core professional practice.

THE CHALLENGES OF CANCER

Cancer diagnosis, investigations and treatment can trigger a rollercoaster of feelings. These can include dread and uncertainty and, despite advances in medical care, deep concerns about the future and the risk of early death may be provoked. The challenges of disease symptoms, treatment side-effects and changes in the ability to carry out normal daily activities can drive individuals to look for support, to fight, withdraw or exist in a constant state of heightened anxiety (Moorey and Greer 2002). These responses may be linked to existing coping strategies and level of illness/treatment burden and prognosis, if known. Reported benefits of complementary therapies provided to people living with cancer include:

- reduction in anxiety, stress, depression and fatigue scores

- increased ability cope with symptoms, such as discomfort and treatment burden

- improvements in the ability to relax and be less fearful

- improvement in the quality and duration of sleep.

If we know that complementary therapies can effect change, this poses the question, 'How can therapists build on this work and promote greater resilience?' A possible answer would be for the therapist to help patients find resources to sustain themselves beyond the therapy session.

WHAT IS RESILIENCE?

Vaillant (1995) has suggested that 'We all know perfectly well what resilience means until we listen to someone else try to define it' (p.284). Concept analysis attempts to provide clarity, insight and understanding by determining the most frequently occurring defining attributes, elements and uses of a given term. The work of Earvolino-Ramirez (2007) identified the following attributes that support our 'intuitive' understanding of what resilience might be and provides a starting point for this chapter (see Table 2.1).

The scientific study of resilience emerged in the 1970s from the study of children who thrived despite extreme hardship or risk (Egeland, Carlson and Sroufe 1993; Luthar, Cicchetti and Becker 2000; Masten 2001). The evolution of research into resilience can be divided into 'waves'. Each wave focuses on particular mechanisms and stimulates further research in how best to foster or promote resilience processes (O'Dougherty-Wright, Masten and Narayan 2013). Contemporary research into resilience now represents a fusion of academic enquiry from fields as diverse as ecosystems (Harris 2011), disaster management (United Nations International Strategy for Disaster Reduction 2011) and psychobiological mechanisms (Charney 2004). The universality of this powerful concept in turn helps to maintain a vibrant, thriving discourse that informs therapeutic application and assessment.

Table 2.1: Attributes which support our 'intuitive'
understanding of what resilience might be

Attribute	Meaning
Rebounding	A sense of bouncing back and moving on
Reintegration	A process after disruption where the experience is assimilated and given a sense of coherence (personal meaning)
High expectancy	A sense of purpose or achievement in life
Self-determination	Encompasses self-worth (a strong internal belief that whatever life brings, the individual can adapt) and self-efficacy to enable the mastery of experiences
Social support	Opportunities for connection and support that are perceived as meaningful to the individual
Connection	A sense of belonging and purpose that protects against isolation, helplessness and hopelessness
Flexibility	The essence of adaptability and rolling with the changes
Sense of humour	This is the only attribute that is shared among every recorded demographic! It helps to reduce the burden of adversity by moderating the intensity of emotional reactions as well as enhancing effective coping mechanisms

RESILIENCE RESEARCH: THE FIRST WAVE

The first wave research generates a useful consensus regarding what is inferred (concluded from the evidence) from the concept of 'resilience' itself. Contemporary understanding of resilience encapsulates the complex and ongoing interaction between: 1) A challenge, disturbance or threat caused by an adverse (potentially harmful) event; and 2) How an individual, a system or community positively adapts/responds to that event.

Self-reflective question 1: *What does the term 'resilience' conjure up for me personally in my own life?*

The first wave particularly emphasizes individual personality traits such as 'stress resistance' and examines the individual's ability or 'competence' in achieving key tasks in stages of development. These include stages such as learning to read, developing friendships or parenting a child (Kraemer *et al.* 2001; Rutter 1985). The language of the researchers is often couched in terms that evoke threat or defence, such as the focus on 'risk' (a measurable variable that can predict a specific, undesirable outcome), 'vulnerability' (the susceptibility to an undesired outcome) and 'protective' (a helpful predictor in situations of difficulty or risk) factors. Despite such terms, the examination of resilience represents an important paradigm shift away from 'deficits' to 'strengths-based' research (Kent and Davis 2010).

> Self-reflective question 2: *How much of my complementary therapy work focuses on identifying and acknowledging the patient's strengths as well his/her presenting problems?*

When having a dialogue with a patient, consider the individual's resources past and present, e.g. the patient's use of music, his/her relationship with nature and memories of being supported and loved, as well as his/her stated problems/concerns.

> Self-reflective question 3: *How does the environment in which I work, for example a hospital/hospice (or somewhere else), potentially promote or inhibit a patient's resilience?*

It is important for the therapist to consider how the clinical environment may inadvertently reinforce the vulnerability and isolation that patients can experience when challenged by a life-threatening diagnosis. For example, it is helpful to pay mindful attention to the air of 'welcome' and the ease of the therapy space. Subtle considerations could include mentioning movement of air from an open window or fan, the comfort of a chair, a pillow placed 'just right' (adjusting it until that is achieved), and providing ample time for patients to make choices and consolidate personal reflection.

Setting up a support group to promote resilience

'Fighting spirit' has been identified as one of the helpful stances taken by people with cancer (Moorey and Greer 2002; Watson *et al.* 1994). When the author set up a weekly mind-body drop-in group session, 'Fighting Spirit' was adopted for the name of the group.

The aim of the group was to offer support to cancer patients, relatives, carers and staff. Therapists trained in hypnotherapy, guided imagery and mindfulness practice facilitated the sessions. There was ample space in the waiting area for people to 'arrive' and connect with each other. It was also noted that patients started to 'go for a chat' after the sessions in the coffee bar provided by the organization. This social activity seemed to reinforce the benefits of the group members' reflective time together. As this became a positive feature of the group, the facilitator suggested that the activity could be an option for all group members.

All the sessions had four 'elements' or themes: 1) Resilience, 2) Supportive Allies, 3) Inner Strength and 4) Enhancing Energy. Participants chose an element for the week and were given time to consider and then document their personal definition of what each element might mean. Additionally, they had the opportunity to give a 'before and after' session rating. Feedback was welcomed in any way that felt meaningful to the participant and was verbal, written, drawn or even sung (thank you, Monty Python!). Importantly, each individual 'chose' an element for themselves, and, at the end of the session, the different elements were woven together to create a personal resilience prescription for the week. In this way, the session both literally and metaphorically supported powerful resilience processes (see Box 2.1).

The four 'elements' provided options for subsequent sessions, allowing the possibility of a four-week programme. The reality of an acute cancer centre is that the group participants often change from week to week; needs may be dependent on what has happened on that day, so being flexible is key (see Chapter 10).

**Box 2.1: Examples taken from patients'
comments about the elements**

- Resilience: Regaining something I feel I have lost in the last few months. I found the session useful as a reminder of what is helpful to let go of and what is strengthening. Thank you. (Male patient)

- Supportive allies: Thank you for this experience. This is the second time I have experienced 'Fighting Spirit' and I have benefited enormously. Ready to face the world. I feel incredibly calm and relaxed. I think I have more allies than I thought I had. I need to spend more time thinking about them. (Female patient)

- Inner Strength: Determination to live life to the full. Tearful. (Female carer)

- Enhancing Energy: I've had a busy day but after this relaxation session I feel more energized than before and very relaxed. (Female staff member)

RESILIENCE RESEARCH: THE SECOND WAVE

The second wave of resilience research emphasizes the unique nature of adversity and the protective processes involving successful adaptation. The development is succinctly described by Masten (2011) as the 'how do people become resilient' question in the resilience research. The process of 'how' is evidenced by close examination of stages of development throughout an individual's life. This 'life course' perspective includes consideration of the importance of biology, family networks, wider cultural, spiritual and other social connections (Cicchetti 2010; Luthar 2006). Attachment styles, self-soothing abilities, neurological development, learning styles, experiences of mastery, self-motivation and personal values are all key variables that are found to powerfully influence development. These aspects of an individual's 'life course' work together to protect an individual, and facilitate recovery or restoration (Masten 2001). Second wave researchers invite us to think in terms of a 'resilience and vulnerability continuum' that reaches across multiple, ever-changing domains, including the physical, psychological, social relationships and job performance (O'Dougherty-Wright *et al.* 2013). The challenge for therapists remains how best to meet the holistic needs of a patient (and/or carer) and to nurture their enduring, adaptive capabilities to promote resilience. The case study below demonstrates how sensitively exploring a patient's background can help to identify resources that have helped the patient through previous difficulties, to create his personal 'stackable images' and maximize resilience. A patient's journey through cancer treatment has the potential to be an additional source of strength for his/her future; if shared, other patients, carers and healthcare professionals could also benefit.

Case study 2.1: Risk, vulnerabilities and building resilience

Alan struggled with feelings of claustrophobia during head and neck radiotherapy and after ten days he refused further treatment. He reported feeling overwhelmed by his fear of suffocation and being alone. Alan revealed that he was the youngest of four children and his mother had been married to an abusive husband. Alan's childhood was disrupted as the family were relocated three times to escape. When gently asked, 'What do you think helps you to cope?' Alan replied that he had promised his mum he would never kill himself. Alan's mum, her resourcefulness and strong protective instincts, reconnected Alan to feelings of belonging, being cared for and caring for others, including a love of animals, particularly of his dog Staffy. Alan recorded his feelings sentence by sentence on his mobile phone – he found this easier because of dyslexia. The list that Alan played 'at difficult times' said:

- I know the value of friendship and love.
- I love nature and animals.
- I have survived a lot of pain.
- I keep my word.

Alan was asked what his mum might have to add the above list. He replied, 'She'd say I love you to bits and you're a good son.' The love of his mum was acknowledged as 'a tower of strength' and he was pleased to add it to his resources. Using these memories and his recorded list, he welcomed support from guided imagery during the radiotherapy procedures and enjoyed receiving massages from the ward therapist. Alan completed his 30 sessions of radiotherapy and took a photograph of his mask to record his achievement (see Figure 1.3).

RESILIENCE RESEARCH: THE THIRD WAVE

Third wave resilience research is characterized by the in-depth analysis of strategic interventions intended to promote 'protective' processes and develop resilience where it is absent or needs enhancing. Examples include the boosting of needed resources, strengthening significant relationships and encouraging bonding with helpful social groups. There is a strong preventative focus that identifies how to reduce the risks of adverse exposure, prevent cumulative trauma and minimize exposure to adversity; the purpose is to maximize a 'positive cascade' resulting from timely, powerful interventions (Patterson, Forgatch and De Garmo 2010). In addition, researchers examine the relevance of the timing and intensity of an intervention, i.e. the 'dose' (Masten and Cicchetti 2010). Ongoing research questions concerned with moderators and mediators are also relevant to therapists working to integrate resilience processes into their practice.

Padesky and Mooney (2012) have devised a 'four-step strengths-based model', which is designed to bring hidden strengths into patient awareness to help build a personal model of resilience. Patient-generated images, particularly their own words and metaphors, are used as potent reminders of their abilities to 'experience resilience' rather than achieve specific outcomes. This is an especially important point, as 'being resilient' does not necessarily translate into feeling positive or optimistic. In practice, this is achieved by searching through the patient's commonplace experiences. A simple question, 'What is the one thing you do every day because you really want to do it?' can elicit determination and problem-solving abilities, in addition to offering nourishing, restorative moments. Once identified, these examples can be used to 'copy and paste' into the person's reflection on current areas of challenge, which can then be tested, tweaked, applied and practised, or even rejected as a strategy.

Case study 2.2: Using nature as a resource

Marjorie was offered guided imagery treatment to help soothe and calm her after she was unable to complete an MRI scan. Marjorie mentioned her irritation at possibly being late home because, 'I'm going to miss my nature programme.' Her therapist immediately noted the opportunity to connect to her motivation and asked her to share what she loved most about these programmes. Marjorie had a particular affinity to elephants and admired their intelligence and playfulness. She described a film where female elephants had worked together to rescue a baby elephant trapped in the mud while the male elephants stood around forming a protective circle. At one point she started to laugh, and immediately pointed out the parallel between herself and what was currently happening. Marjorie's capacity for humour, imagination and connection helped her identify with a sense of protection and guidance. The therapist immediately recognized how he could help Marjorie to utilize her strengths; he enabled a connection with Marjorie's innate resilience, collapsed the fear and Marjorie successfully completed the scan. Marjorie also reported counting elephants and giving each of them names, helping the time to pass more quickly. After Marjorie's treatment had been completed, she made a gift to the complementary therapy team of two beautifully decorated elephants. They adorn the office and serve as visual metaphors for the whole team to enjoy.

Case study 2.3: Accessing resilience through stillness

Niamh was waiting for the first dose of chemotherapy and was anxious about cannulation. She was very frightened and her partner described her state as being 'shit scared' and he was fed up with 'listening to that bloody CD she bought'. The therapist decided that it would be more helpful if Niamh were to have a treatment away from the chemotherapy unit. She involved another therapist to use the HEARTS approach with her so there could be one person holding Niamh's head and one holding her feet. The two therapists sat with Niamh for 20 minutes while she closed her eyes and relaxed. (The therapists were very relaxed as well!)

During the last five minutes, the therapist holding Niamh's head invited her to think about what would she would like to leave behind in the room, and what would be useful on her visit to the chemotherapy unit.

When Niamh returned to an alert state she said, 'I will take the memory of your hands on my head and feet...I don't feel so alone in all this any more.' She 'sailed through chemotherapy' thinking about booking in for another 'many-handed session'. The CD, however, was never played again. Niamh had made her choice about what was helpful; she rejected something that was not a resource for her.

Although beyond the remit of this chapter, there has been significant development in our scientific understanding of resilience. We can now appreciate that resilience occurs at multiple levels, such as within the cell's genetic code or gene expression. Resilience even impacts on the 'plasticity' of the ever-changing brain. Mindfulness techniques and a deeper understanding of attachment theory can enable our patients to learn how to physically and neurologically 'rewire'. This is achieved most efficiently by modelling and teaching self-soothing and emotional regulation (a process by which individuals can influence and reduce the intensity of their distress). We look forward to 'groundbreaking research' that supports what we instinctively know already – that the therapeutic relationship and the relaxation response are powerful tools for healing (Roemer, Williston and Rollins 2015).

Self-reflective question 4: *Should therapists assist patient and carers in building resilience in the face of current and future challenges?*

Perhaps this is the most important question to ask. In working with issues such as anxiety, distress and panic, therapists can explore and build a toolbox of resourceful therapeutic techniques and approaches to offer to patients. Promoting resilience may seem to be a new role for some therapists; however, it could be beneficial if the therapist came to a situation with a willingness to assist an individual in uncovering resources. There is empowerment through offering the patient choice while respecting the right of the individual to refuse, acknowledging that saying 'No' is a success. Rejecting an intervention(s) is an assertion of choice and can deepen the therapeutic work, for example by suggesting, 'You know you don't want massage at the moment…but you said the other techniques might be more useful.'

Of course, it could be argued that complementary therapists are there just to provide a relaxing massage, without any expectations beyond the treatment. However, a patient will often talk to a therapist as he/she moves into a relaxed state, providing an opportunity to engage with resilience work on a deeper therapeutic level. Giving a patient an aromastick is more than a takeaway present; it can be a potent reminder of a deeply relaxing session, a time which one patient described as 'being on holiday from cancer'. Supporting a patient to utilize an aromastick when managing a challenging situation requires making the process overt, rather than simply hoping it might happen (see Chapter 8).

SUMMARY

This book contains numerous suggestions and adaptations to practice, which contribute to identifying a variety ways of building resilience. The world is literally our oyster. Providing the right conditions to access what feels right for a patient includes:

- listening

- identifying allies

- making choices and rejecting some

- anchoring what feels right

- stacking the allies and resources.

REFERENCES

Baker, B. S., Harrington, J. E., Choi, B.S. Kropf, P., Muller, I. and Hoffman, C. J. (2012) 'A randomized controlled pilot feasibility study of the physical and psychological effects of an integrated support program in breast cancer.' *Complementary Therapies in Clinical Practice 18*, 3, 182–189.

Cicchetti, D. (2010) 'Resilience under conditions of extreme stress: A multilevel perspective.' *World Psychiatry, 9,* 3, 145–154.

Charney, D. (2004) 'Psychobiological mechanisms of resilience and vulnerability: implications for successful adaptation to extreme stress.' *American Journal of Psychiatry 161,* 2, 195–216.

Earvolino-Ramirez, M. (2007) 'Resilience: a concept analysis.' *Nursing Forum 42,* 2, 73–82.

Egeland, B., Carlson, E., Sroufe, L.A. (1993) 'Resilience as process.' *Development and Psychopathology 5,* 4, 517–528.

Harris, K. (2011) 'Resilience in Practice: Operationalizing the Ten Characteristics of Resilience through the Case of Greening Darfur. Strengthening Climate Resilience.' Discussion Paper 10, Institute of Development Studies: Brighton.

Kent, M. and Davis, M.C. (2010) 'Resilience Interventions: The Emergence of Capacity-Building Programs and Models.' In J. W. Reich, A. J. Zautra, and J. S. Hall (eds) *Handbook Of Adult Resilience.* London: The Guildford Press.

Kraemer, H.C. Stice, E. Kazdin, A.E. Offord, D.R. *et al.* (2001) 'How do risk factors work together? Mediators, moderators, and independent, overlapping, and proxy risk factors.' *American Journal of Psychiatry 158,* 6, 848–856.

Kutner, J. S., Smith, M. C., Corbin, L., Hemphill, L. et al. (2008) 'Massage therapy versus simple touch to Improve pain and mood in patients with advanced cancer: a randomized trial.' *Annals of Internal Medicine 149,* 6, 369–379.

Luthar, S. S. (2006) 'Resilience in Development: A Synthesis of Research Across Five Decades.' In D. Cicchetti and D. Cohen (eds) *Developmental Psychopathology: Risk, Disorder, and Adaptation.* New York: Wiley.

Luthar, S.S., Cicchetti, D., Becker, B. (2000) 'The construct of resilience: a critical evaluation and guidelines for future work.' *Child Development 71,* 3, 543–562.

Masten, A.S. (2001) 'Ordinary magic: resilience processes in development.' *American Psychologist 56*, 3, 227–238.

Masten, A.S. and Cicchetti, D. (2010) 'Editorial: Developmental cascades [Special Issue, Part 1].' *Development and Psychopathology 22*, 3, 491–495.

Masten, A.S. (2011) 'Resilience in children threatened by extreme adversity: Frameworks for research, practice, and translational synergy.' *Development and Psychopathology 23*, 2, 493–506.

Moorey, S. and Greer, S. (2002) *Cognitive Behaviour Therapy for People with Cancer.* Oxford: Oxford University Press.

O'Dougherty-Wright, M., Masten, A.S., Narayan, A.J. (2013) 'Resilience Processes in Development: Four Waves of Research on Positive Adaptation in the Context of Adversity.' In S. Goldstein and R.B. Brooks (eds) *Handbook of Resilience In Children.* New York: Springer.

Padesky, C.A. and Mooney, K.A. (2012) 'Strengths-based cognitive behavioural therapy: A four-step model to build resilience.' *Clinical Psychology and Psychotherapy 19*, 4, 283–290.

Patterson, G.R., Forgatch, M.S., DeGarmo, D.S. (2010) 'Cascading effects following intervention.' *Development and Psychopathology 22*, 4, 941–970.

Roemer, L., Williston, S.K., Rollins, L. G. (2015) 'Mindfulness and emotion regulation.' *Current Opinion in Psychology 3*, 52–57.

Rutter, M. (1985) 'Resilience in the face of adversity – Protective factors and resistance to psychiatric disorder.' *The British Journal of Psychiatry 147*, 6, 598–611.

Smith, M. C., Kemp, J., Hemphill, L. and Vojir, C.P. (2002) 'Outcomes of therapeutic massage for hospitalized cancer patients.' *Journal of Nursing Scholarship 34*, 3, 257–262.

United Nations International Strategy for Disaster Reduction (2011) *Global Assessment Report on Disaster Risk Reduction: Revealing Risk, Redefining Development.* UNISDR. Available at www.preventionweb.net/english/hyogo/gar/2011/en/home/download.html, accessed on 12 February 2016.

Vaillant, G.E. (1995) *The Wisdom Of The Ego.* London: Harvard University Press.

Watson, M., Law, M., Santos, M., Greer, S. (1994) 'The Mini-MAC: Further Development of the Adjustment to Cancer Scale.' *Journal of Psychosocial Oncology, 12*, 3, 33–46.

Chapter 3

THE RESOURCEFUL THERAPIST

Ann Carter and Dr Peter A. Mackereth

KEY WORDS

therapists, roles, skills, challenges, supervision, reflection

INTRODUCTION

For many therapists working to support cancer patients and their carers, the medical world can be both a confusing and rewarding one. Most therapists quickly come to the realization that the techniques and skills learnt in their initial training need either adapting or are insufficient to meet the complex needs of this setting. Importantly, therapists need to become familiar with the environment, safety issues and understanding of cancer and its treatments, as well as feeling confident when communicating with a wide group of healthcare professionals. Additionally, therapists in cancer care settings will have physical, emotional and spiritual responses to what they see, hear, smell, touch and intuitively feel. This chapter is about therapists developing the resources to be fit for cancer care practice. The content will also explore some of the factors involved in helping therapists to stay resourceful and effective and to value their work.

THERAPISTS' BACKGROUNDS

Although complementary therapists are an emerging and evolving workforce, there is limited information about how they are trained and supported in acute cancer care practice. Mackereth *et al.* (2009a) investigated the motivation of therapists (n=51) working in cancer care across three sites, including a hospital, a cancer care day service and a hospice. Most of the participants reported having experience of cancer (or another serious illness) within the family, or with a friend, and had a desire to make a difference by offering complementary therapies (CTs). Six out of 18 of the participants had made a career change from nursing, in part projected by paperwork and lack of contact with patients. Many had diverse professional backgrounds and had embarked on their second or third careers; some were providing therapies as volunteers or as work experience.

In a second paper, Mackereth *et al.* (2009b) explored therapists' training in cancer care, concluding that there is a need for ongoing professional development and standardization of training, which includes courses, support and supervision.

In a third study, Mackereth *et al.* (2010) explored the rewards and challenges of therapists (n=15) working in cancer care settings and the role of supervision through focus group interviews. Participants valued their work, and reported that providing CTs in cancer care was of itself rewarding, empowering and a privilege.

THERAPISTS' ROLES

Therapists' roles can vary widely depending on their skills and the expectations of the organization. CTs are increasingly being used alongside conventional cancer treatments to support patients undergoing chemotherapy and radiotherapy (Baker *et al.* 2012). Research suggests there are beneficial psychological effects for patients attending for cancer treatment, lowering levels of anxiety, worry and depression (Billhult *et al.* 2009; Kutner *et al.* 2008). Utilizing CTs to assist with specific symptoms, such as nausea and pain, has also been investigated (Cassileth, Trevisan and Gubili 2007). Patients and carers are very appreciative of complementary therapists providing interventions during hospitalization (Shorofi 2011; Smith *et al.* 2002). An area of emerging practice for therapists is helping patients during medical procedures and treatments, such as intravenous cannulation, complex invasive radiotherapy procedures and having dressings changed.

FULFILLING THE ROLE

Four key areas need to be addressed in developing as a resourceful therapist in cancer care, particularly during the acute phase of the patient's investigations, procedures and treatment. These include:

- being able to recognize emotional needs which could be contained and eased throughout a procedure or medical treatment

- feeling comfortable and open to supporting patients and carers during treatments and medical procedures, such as a scan or cannulation

- being able to learn and then teach self-soothing techniques, so that patients have a resource to utilize during future procedures and challenging situations

- recognizing that carers also require support during the patient's procedures and that they will benefit from help to manage their own stressors (see Chapter 14).

Typically, therapists train to offer distinct therapies within a private therapy space and may have little exposure to delivering treatments within wards, clinics and in public areas of a hospital or hospice. A therapist's induction requires familiarity and awareness of safety concerns around equipment, emergency call systems, infection control processes (for example, hand washing, isolation procedures), as well as a working knowledge of cancer, treatments and side-effects (see Chapter 1). Practical mandatory training such as fire, first aid and moving and handling is usually delivered as classroom sessions. Increasingly, topics such as confidentiality, safeguarding, duty of care and equality and diversity are delivered via online training. Importantly, to function safely and effectively within an acute setting, therapists need a period of internship, supervized by an experienced therapist, with opportunities to observe and engage in paired working, and time to evaluate activities and the experience. Implicit in delivering CTs within an acute, supportive and palliative care role are the following aspects of patient care. According to Mackereth and Carter (2006), therapists need to:

- adapt the therapies they practise to suit the needs of individuals, so they act in a helping and supportive role

- acknowledge boundaries in terms of their knowledge and skills to themselves and others

- recognize that the role is concerned with working 'on the edge' of complementary therapy practice, while at the same time finding safe and creative ways of working

- respect a patient's autonomy and his/her right to refuse treatment

- work within an ethical framework, acknowledging a 'duty of care'

- be prepared to evaluate the outcomes of their work

- have an understanding of the organization's complementary therapy policy and any standard operating procedures.

THE EMOTIONAL SIDE OF WORKING AS A COMPLEMENTARY THERAPIST

In addition to the practical side of working as a complementary therapist in cancer care settings, there are also emotional and spiritual issues, which can arise from the work (see Chapter 15). Similar concerns preoccupy other health professionals in cancer care and include:

- taking thoughts about an individual's circumstances home, cognitively and emotionally

- feeling helpless that the therapist could not do more for the patient or carer

- experiencing bereavement; dealing with loss when a patient dies or is discharged

- supporting a distressed patient, for example helping with a particularly unpleasant procedure, or where malodour is present (see Chapter 9)

- attempting to meet everyone else's needs at the expense of one's own; this is sometimes known as the 'compassion trap'

- being aware of triggers that remind the therapist of their own cancer experiences, losses and bereavement(s).

There is a need for therapists to nurture their own bodies and spirit and to look after their own needs. For some, this may involve a regular meditation or mindfulness practice, receiving a complementary therapy, or spending time doing something totally different and enjoyable (see Case study 3.1). One of the key ways of supporting therapists is to support their professional and emotional development through supervision (including mentoring), reflective practice and through education, for example training courses.

Case study 3.1: Understanding bereavement

David, a volunteer therapist, worked in a hospice. In part, he wanted to 'put something back' after the loss of his partner. A year into his role, David worked with a patient who was dying with the same cancer as that of his partner. After three sessions he began to 'take the situation home', ruminating over how he could help 'fix things' for the patient and family. In supervision, David shared that these feelings and his own loss were overwhelming and he was wondering about asking another therapist to take over. The supervisor explored what it was about the patient that triggered the connection. Through talking, David realized that he was investing too much in the outcome if the sessions, rather than 'being with the patient' and recognizing that his own losses were separate and personal to him. David decided to continue working with the patient, but asked to share the treatments with another therapist. He also started to plan a memorial event for his partner and recommenced with attending weekly tai chi classes.

SUPERVISION

Supervision is a process which helps therapists to become more confident and able to deal with situations they find challenging. Stone (2010) suggests that supervision should be seen as a safeguard for competent and safe practice. Ideally, the supervisor and the supervisee should meet at regular intervals to discuss matters that may arise during the supervisee's work (Mackereth and Carter 2006). For the process to be effective and welcomed, it must be perceived as useful, safe and relevant to the supervisee's practice (Mackereth 2000). See Figure 3.1.

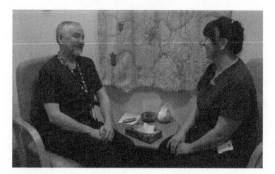

*Figure 3.1: Supervision sessions can be both enjoyable and
a useful tool in developing skills and resolving challenges*

There is no statutory requirement for complementary therapists to have supervision; however, there are several ways it can be offered within an organization, or, at the discretion of the therapist, outside the organization. Some suggestions are given in Box 3.1.

Box 3.1: Optional supervision methods

- One-to-one: one supervisor to one supervisee (as in Figure 3.1 above) meeting regularly.
- The complementary therapy co-ordinator/clinical lead/ manager organizes group supervision for his/her own team. (A shortcoming of this approach is that some therapists won't want to discuss anything of a personal nature as they might be judged by their peer group or manager.)
- A member of staff not directly connected with complementary therapies offers supervision.
- Supervision can be practised in short sessions with a specific objective, for example 'the need to speak about...'
- Therapists organize their own supervision outside the organization, on either a one-to-one or group basis.

REFLECTIVE PRACTICE

One of the most resourceful skills that a therapist can acquire is the ability to practise reflection, either through supervision or as a process to use on an individual basis, or with a colleague. We have found Johns's (1993) Model of Reflection to be particularly useful (see Box 3.2). Other options of reflective practice models have been devised by Gibbs (1988) and Atkins and Murphy (1994).

Box 3.2: An outline of a model of reflection based on Johns's model (2004)

Please note: depending on the situation, some aspects of this model may not be directly relevant or there may be some overlap with another component in a different section.

1. Motivation to be involved in the reflection
- Why would it be helpful for me to reflect and review this event?

2. Reviewing the event
- What was the event as it happened?
- What factors were contributing to this event at the time?
- Were there any other relevant background factors to my experience?

3. Reflecting
- When I was involved in the event, what did I want to achieve?
- What factors influenced my actions?
- What were the consequences for myself, patients, colleagues?
- How did I feel as the event unfolded?
- What did my colleagues feel about the experience?
- How do I know that was how they felt?

4. Alternatives
- What other courses of action did I have at the time?
- Had I chosen to do something else, what might have been the outcome?
- What stopped me from doing something differently?

5. What have I learned?
- Faced with a similar situation, what would I do now?
- How could I have been more effective?
- What have I learned from reviewing the event?
- How do I feel now about the event?

6. Application
- How has this process helped my development as a therapist?

BOUNDARIES AND THERAPEUTIC RELATIONSHIPS

In terms of therapeutic relationships, Stone (2008) refers to the limits of the professional relationship. This can be a difficult area for some therapists, especially when they feel that they haven't 'done enough', or they could help the patient more if the friendship was more 'friendly'. According to the Council for Health and Regulatory Excellence (CHRE) (2008) it is the responsibility of the professional person to set and maintain clear boundaries. Therapists have found Campbell's (1984) analogy, useful in terms of 'framing' the professional relationship as a 'companion' and in allowing patients to 'make their own journey' when the treatment is concluded, to be useful. Campbell (1984) suggests that this companionship emerges through meaningful contact and ceases when the 'joint purpose' comes to conclusion. The 'good companion' shares freely, without imposing, allowing the patient or carer to make their 'own journey'.

Another challenge which therapists may find difficult is wanting to 'fix it' for the patient or feeling inadequate when he/she has not been able to effect the change they wanted for the patient (see Box 3.3). Thinking over the events of the day, questioning and replaying interactions over and over again can interfere with family and leisure time. A useful metaphor originates from Blanchard, Onken and Burrows (1989), the essence of which is outlined in Box 3.3. The 'monkeys' are symbols of people's problems.

DEVELOPING THE THERAPIST'S ROLE IN TERMS OF SKILLS

As well as supporting therapists in terms of personal development and increasing confidence, it is also important to help them to develop their skills base. This will enable them to offer a wider range of options to the patient and will help to develop a professional approach. Additional skills which complementary therapists find useful include relaxation techniques, guided imagery, breathing techniques, skills for stress management, HEARTS, aromasticks and the resourceful use of language. We have found all of these approaches useful for therapists to combine with existing therapeutic skills where the situation requires their use.

Box 3.3: Leaving work behind, or how to manage monkeys

Everyone has pet monkeys, and all monkeys need to be fed and watered overnight.

Monkeys need to be looked after until they can be gently persuaded to take a holiday, or to leave home and find something more purposeful to do. Kind and caring people love to look after monkeys. Of course, they have their own pet monkeys to look after, and to feed and water overnight...but they also have a tendency to attract more monkeys, which don't belong to them. These 'extra' monkeys are gathered up like a monkey family throughout the day, and taken to the therapist's home at night, where they are very well attended to.

We all need to remember that gathering up other people's monkeys is a time-consuming occupation. Monkeys will be just as happy being fed and watered by their original owners without therapists taking them home and looking after them.

So maybe it's best if we support people in looking after their own monkeys for the time we spend with them – then they go home with their monkeys and we go home with ours.

INNOVATION AND LEADERSHIP

Another area for development is innovation and leadership. Some therapists will be very happy to come in to the organization, see patients and then to go home, feeling satisfied with their work. Others will want more, and may be looking to develop their role, for example in managing others and teaching and contributing to the service through creativity (see Case studies 3.2 and 3.3).

Case study 3.2: A pivotal moment

Barbara, a therapist in beauty therapy, attended a course on HEARTS out of curiosity. During an experience of receiving HEARTS as a participant, she came to the realization that that this way of being in touch with people was powerful and it awoke in her a desire to change careers. Barbara became a volunteer and attended further training, so she could add additional therapies to her toolbox. Within eight years of making this major career change, she worked as a senior therapist, managed her own clinic, contributed to publications, became involved in teaching and then became a centre co-ordinator.

Case study 3.3: Being creative to support patients

Frustrated with justified health and safety concerns around using an electric aromatic diffuser, Jan proposed to create 'aroma pots' which could be used in a side room to assist with malodours. With help from colleagues, various blends were created. Cottonwool was placed within a small screw-topped disposable container which absorbed the blend (see Chapter 9). Through monitoring and feedback from staff, patients and carers, a protocol evolved that included a daily review of the blend and its use, an information sheet and a rapid process of referral to ensure that malodour was tackled as soon as possible. The team also established communication with the tissue viability staff and infection control to explore suitable dressings and a role for essential oils.

SUMMARY

This chapter has addressed some of the main areas which could support therapists in 'staying resourceful'. It has highlighted the need for supporting therapists in developing their toolboxes, both in terms of delivering complementary therapies and working in clinical settings. Some of the motivation for working in cancer care has been covered and we would like to emphasize the benefits of a comprehensive induction programme, supervision and the use of reflective practice. We have acknowledged that therapists may need help with establishing boundaries and managing the stressors that they may experience. We also recognize that some therapists will be pleased to contribute more to the service, if given the opportunity.

REFERENCES

Atkins, S. and Murphy, K. (1994) 'Reflective Practice.' *Nursing Standard 8*, 39, 49–56.

Billhult, A., Lindholm, C., Gunnarsson, R., Stener-Victorin, E. (2009) 'The effect of massage on immune function and stress in women with breast cancer – a randomized controlled trial.' *Autonomic Neuroscience: Basic and Clinical 150*, 1–2, 111–115.

Blanchard, K., Oncken Jr. W., Burrows H. (1989) *The One Minute Manager Meets the Monkey.* London: William Morrow and Company.

Campbell A.V. (1984) *Moderated Love: a Theology of Professional Care.* London: SPCK Publishing.

Cassileth, B., Trevisan, C., Gubili, J. (2007) 'Complementary therapies for cancer pain.' *Current Pain and Headache Report 11*, 4, 265–269.

Council for Health and Regulatory Excellence (2008) 'Clear sexual boundaries between healthcare professionals and patients: responsibilities of healthcare professionals.' Available at www.professionalstandards.org.uk/docs/default-source/publications/policy-advice/sexual-boundaries-responsibilities-of-healthcare-professionals-2008.pdf?sfvrsn=6, accessed on 12 February 2016.

Gibbs, G. (1988) *Learning by Doing: A Guide to Teaching and Learning Methods.* Oxford: Oxford Polytechnic Further Education Unit.

Johns, C. (1993) 'Achieving Effective Work as a Professional Activity.' In J.E. Schober, and S.M. Hinchliff (eds) *Towards Advanced Nursing Practice* (1995). London: Arnold.

Mackereth, P. (2000) 'Clinical Supervision and Complementary Therapies.' In D. Rankin-Box (ed.) *Nurses' Handbook of Complementary Therapies.* London: Churchill Livingstone.

Mackereth, P. and Carter, A. (2006) 'Professional and Potent Practice.' In: P. Mackereth and A Carter (eds) *Massage and Bodywork: Adapting Therapies for Cancer Care.* London: Elsevier.

Mackereth, P., Carter. A., Parkin. S, Stringer, J. *et al.* (2009a) 'Complementary therapists' motivation to work in cancer/supportive and palliative care: a multi-centre case study.' *Complementary Therapies in Clinical Practice 15,* 3, 161–165.

Mackereth, P., Carter, A., Parkin, S., Stringer, J. *et al.* (2009b) 'Complementary therapists' training and cancer care: A multi-site study.' *European Journal of Oncology Nursing 13,* 3, 330–335.

Mackereth, P., Parkin, S., Donald, G., Antcliffe, N. (2010) 'Clinical supervision and complementary therapists: An exploration of the rewards and challenges of cancer care.' *Complementary Therapies in Clinical Practice 16,* 3, 143–148.

Shorofi, S. (2011) 'Complementary and alternative medicine (CAM) among hospitalised patients: reported use of CAM and reasons for use, CAM preferred during hospitalisation, and the socio-demographic determinants of CAM users.' *Complementary Therapies in Clinical Practice 17,* 4, 199–205.

Stone, J. (2008) 'Respecting professional boundaries: what CAM practitioners need to know.' *Complementary Therapies in Clinical Practice 14,* 1, 2–7.

Stone, J. (2010) 'Professional, Ethical and Legal Issues in Hypnotherapy.' In A. Cawthorn and P.A. Mackereth (eds) *Integrative Hypnotherapy, Complementary Approaches in Clinical Care.* London: Elsevier.

Chapter 4

EFFECTIVE DOCUMENTATION

Ann Carter and Dr Peter A. Mackereth

KEY WORDS

policy, standard operating procedures, documentation,
patients' notes, benchmarking, audit

INTRODUCTION

Complementary therapy services in cancer care are neither universally accessible nor have agreed standards of care. Pockets of excellence exist with efforts focused on the day-to-day delivery of therapies. The service is often provided by paid sessional workers and, more commonly, by volunteer therapists. Co-ordinators/clinical leads may take responsibility for the delivery of the service; responsibilities normally include developing any documentation necessary to function both safely and effectively within a wider organization such as a hospice or acute cancer care centre.

This chapter examines the importance and benefits of writing, producing and agreeing 'documentation' which supports the delivery and evaluation of the complementary therapy service in the best interest of therapists and patients. Documentation can include an overarching complementary therapy policy (CTP), accompanying standard operating procedures (SOPs) and processes of audit and evaluation. The documentation of treatments in patients' notes/electronic records is also covered in detail.

THE BENEFITS OF POLICIES AND STANDARD OPERATING PROCEDURES (SOPS)

Documentation which supports quality service delivery requires careful consideration and may appear daunting and time-consuming to write. This is particularly true for a new service, or where an existing service is being formalized and integrated fully within wider patient services, for example in an acute cancer centre. Importantly, it could be argued that a robust policy gives credibility to the professionalism that underpins the delivery and acceptance of the complementary therapy service (Fearon 2006). Additionally, it is useful to allocate time and resources to auditing documentation. The outcomes of an audit help to evaluate service effectiveness and support changes that can improve service delivery and the best use of resources.

Tavares (2005, p.4) describes policies as 'agreed rules made by an organization to ensure safe and consistent practice and to manage risk'. Policies are normally written at management level and usually include processes which will lead to optimum professionalism and safety in the delivery of the service. The complementary therapy policy will need to be written in the 'house style' of existing policies, so that it is consistent with the layout which has been approved and owned by the organization.

Given the uniqueness of organizations, it is challenging to offer a 'one size fits all' template for any CTP. Suggestions for inclusions in a policy are given in Box 4.1. Sections of policies may be written at different times during service development, and it is likely that many policies are written to formalize and/or to integrate the different aspects of an existing complementary therapy service. When a policy has been written before a service has commenced, it is likely that the policy will need to be revised during the first few weeks or months to reflect unforeseen situations once the service is in operation.

Sometimes there is confusion between a complementary therapy policy and standard operating procedures (the latter are sometimes referred to as protocols). SOPs contain details for ensuring that the content of the policy is incorporated into everyday practice. They are often descriptions of safe practice, which relate directly to a therapist's work with patients. SOPs can also be written for a range of processes and treatments which form the basis of the complementary therapy service, for example referral processes, one-to-one sessions with patients, and group activities, such as relaxation groups (see Chapter 10).

Box 4.1: Areas of service delivery which could be included in a complementary therapy service policy

- the aim(s) of the complementary therapy service and the target groups to which it applies
- the therapies offered and their evidence base
- the maintenance of a register of therapists, for example a record of current qualifications, insurance, membership of professional bodies and essential checks, such as criminal record checks
- therapist recruitment, interviews and induction processes
- processes for terminating employment/honorary contract or volunteer service
- patient confidentiality and consent processes
- professional boundaries/conflicts of interest; for example, therapists should not promote private practice, the receiving of gifts
- the process by which patients (and carers) can access complementary therapies
- patient assessment and documentation
- access to patients' records
- complaints procedure
- incident reporting
- recording of treatment activity, for example maintaining databases
- hygiene/infection control
- criteria for the introduction of new therapies
- standards for audit
- equality and diversity issues
- mandatory education/training, for example basic life support and manual handling
- review date.

It can be the responsibility of the complementary therapy co-ordinator (CTC) or clinical lead to write both the CTP and the SOPs. Sometimes, the person who takes on the responsibility for this task is another healthcare professional who is designated as the 'lead' for the complementary therapy service. He/she may not be a complementary therapist. In this chapter, the person who has responsibility for the CTP and the SOPs will be referred to as the 'complementary therapy lead' (CT lead).

THE ROLE OF A POLICY

For anyone who is new to writing a policy, this task can be a challenging prospect. Policies cannot be completed overnight and will usually require formal consultation and participation from colleagues in other areas of service management. Other relevant stakeholders may need to be involved, such as patient and service user representatives. Sometimes, policy writing is regarded as a chore; however, producing a policy does have some benefits.

The benefits of either writing a new policy, or updating an existing one are as follows:

- The activity involved in writing a policy facilitates a 'thinking through' of the issues and processes involved in running a service. A service which is fully integrated into patient care will reflect collaboration with other services and existing policies, and this will be demonstrated in the policy, for example links to health and safety, human resources, clinical governance.

- There are opportunities to liaise with other services with which the CT lead may not routinely have direct contact, such as estates, or pharmacy in relationship to the storage and disposal of essential oils.

- Policies that include a referenced evidence base offer opportunities to dispel some of the myths which surround complementary therapies, for example safety concerns relating to chemotherapy and physical contact.

- The policy demonstrates congruence with the existing practices of other services within the organization, thereby enhancing credibility for the service, for example health and safety issues, referral processes and complaints.

- Given the wide variations in therapist training and standards of practice, a policy can provide 'in-house' standards by which therapists will be recruited, for example recognizable and insurable qualification(s).

When writing a policy, drafts will need to be circulated at different stages of the policy's development for consultation. It is helpful if a time limit for review of the document being circulated is stated and adhered to. We recommend that policy drafts are also circulated to therapists so they have the opportunity to review and comment on the content.

Once the policy is agreed, we advise that its implementation is continuously monitored, with any concerns raised at the earliest stage. It is important to recognize that a policy, and indeed any document, can be withdrawn and/or revised should it not comprise best practice. All policies should have a future date for an official review; both internal and external regulations and evidence-based practice may change over time.

THE ROLE OF STANDARD OPERATING PROCEDURES

It is useful to understand the differences between policies and standard operating procedures. SOPs describe in detail how a process is to be carried out; it is directly relevant to patient-facing practice and activities. Policies present 'a bigger picture'. For example, a policy entry may state, 'All therapists are required to make an initial assessment of the patient before the complementary therapy is given' whereas SOPs would describe in detail how the assessment would take place.

An example of an SOP that relates to the documentation of aromatherapy treatments is outlined in Box 4.2.

It is essential that the CT lead explains the processes and the purposes of SOPs to therapists, either on a one-to-one basis or at a therapists' meeting. It is helpful to engage therapists in their understanding of the content of SOPs and how they relate to their practice in the organization. Given that many therapists require training and supervision to work safely in clinical and/or supportive care settings, SOPs provide a useful resource in working collaboratively with the multidisciplinary team. For example, a therapist might be asked to see a patient with acute anxiety related to chemotherapy, who is also living with a long-standing mental health diagnosis. The SOP would advise collaboration with the mental health team (or psycho-oncology) to ensure the best 'joined-up' care.

Box 4.2: An example of a standard operating procedure for documenting complementary therapy treatments

Purpose

This SOP describes the process and the detail required for documenting complementary therapy treatments.

Scope

This SOP applies to the recording of a one-to-one aromatherapy treatment. (The procedure for giving a massage treatment is given in a separate SOP.) Responsibilities of the therapists:

- Before treatment can begin, the therapist must sign the signature bank at the front of the patient's notes the first time he/she works with a patient (if this is standard procedure in the organization).

- The therapist must record a case history on one of the forms provided. The information contained in the case history will inform the approach to the treatment he/she will offer to the patient. The case history will be kept in the patient's notes.

- The therapist must inform the patient about the length of the treatment and details of what it will entail before treatment is commenced, in order to obtain informed consent.

- The patient will sign the case history form which verifies that he/she has given the information to the therapist.

- At the end of the treatment, the therapist must complete the patient's record form. This will include the full date, the time of day and a brief description of the treatment given.

- The names of the essential oils and bases used must be stated in full, for example lavender, bergamot, grapeseed oil. The dose must be stated in terms of the number of drops given and the amount of base oil(s) used. The volume of the base oil should be stated in mls.

- This record of treatment must be signed by the therapist using the signature used in the signature bank.

- Where a patient returns to the organization for further treatment, after the initial course of treatment has been completed, either a second case history must be taken or the original case history must be updated. (The original case history cannot be used for subsequent courses of treatment.)

'LEGAL' PATIENT DOCUMENTATION

All patient notes, whether electronic or a paper copy, are potentially legal documents. Aside from being integral to recording the complementary therapy treatment a patient receives, they also form part of an ongoing therapeutic contract. If documentation does not exist, then an external party has no evidence of what took place (Stone 2010). Inevitably, memory of the events can become distorted over time, and may not be sufficient to satisfy enquiries or an investigation into what happened during a treatment. Patients can request, either informally or formally, to see their notes at any time. Where there is a complaint or dispute between the organization and the patient, or the patient's family, a solicitor can request to see all of the notes relating to patient care, even though the case does not relate directly to complementary therapy treatments. Notes must be written up within 24 hours of the treatment taking place; they must be kept for seven years and they are still legally valid and relevant even if the patient has died. Therapists need to write notes which are clear and concise; abbreviations should not be used unless clarified in the text. Healthcare professionals who are not complementary therapists will need to understand the treatment that the patient has received. Ideally, a patient's treatment notes should be written up as soon as the treatment is over and the record is still fresh in the therapist's memory.

Although both the CTP and the SOPs will have stated the requirements for clear documentation relating to treatments, therapists need to adhere the steps described in the SOPs document. Guidance and supervision of patient record-keeping needs to be a key part of the induction of any new therapist. CT leads need to be assured that therapists are maintaining records that are accurate, relevant, clear, legible and concise, avoiding making judgments and assumptions.

HOW EFFECTIVE ARE POLICIES AND SOPS IN PRACTICE?

Once written and agreed, completed documents such as policies and SOPs may 'end up' being stored either in a file, or they may continue to be referred to, but without any further review taking place. When a review occurs on the allocated date, it is helpful that some evaluation takes place to assess how effective and useful the documentation is on an operational level.

If the contents of the CTP and SOPs are not being followed, then the time spent in preparation of the documents and explaining the contents to therapists is not productive. It is part of the role of the CT lead to explore what is not happening and the reasons why the protocols are not being adhered to. An example is given in Case study 4.1.

Case study 4.1: Are the policies/SOPs being followed in practice?

Sue, a massage therapist, had worked in an organization for two afternoons a week for many years. During a review of notes, it was discovered that Sue was only recording the patient's name and the date of the massage given, without any evidence of an initial case history, details of the treatment or any patient feedback from previous sessions.

When the CT lead asked Sue why she was not following the SOP, she replied, 'My treatments are gentle and I do the same lovely treatment for everyone, so I can't see the point in recording the same thing every week.'

To ensure that the processes and procedures in the SOPs are being followed, and also to help identify training and development needs of therapists (and healthcare professionals) a cyclical audit offers an effective way of evaluating the CTP and SOPS. Murphy (2009) acknowledges that auditing a complementary therapy service can be time-consuming, but importantly it can set complementary therapies on an equal footing with other patient services.

FINDING OUT HOW WELL YOUR POLICY/SOPS ARE WORKING

The following approach has been found to be useful and effective and is outlined in Figure 4.1.

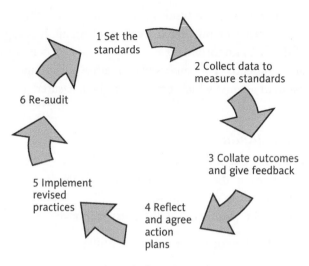

Figure 4.1: The flow of an audit process

WHY SET STANDARDS?

Given that provision of complementary therapies varies across organizations and regions, it could be argued that complementary therapy is still evolving 'best standards of care'. In the UK, the Department of Health *Essence of Care* document (DoH 2010) was launched to help all health professionals take a patient-focused approach to care and to provide assurance that the care is the best it can be. In this document 'benchmarking' was described as, 'a systematic process in which current practice and care are compared to, and amended to attain, best practice and care' (DoH 2010, p.9). The challenge for complementary therapy is to compare its practices with other centres or similar services in the same organization, such as counselling.

Benchmarking quality standards should be an integral part of all CTPs/SOPs and ideally included when the policy is written (Warren, Freer and Molinari 2011). However, SOPs are often written before a policy is completed as they refer to everyday practice, when immediate guidance for therapists' practice is needed. Whatever the timescale, the standards need to reflect the policy contents and other processes which take place within the organization.

Although it is possible to write standards for every single area of the policy, it will never be possible to evaluate them all. It is suggested that some of the most important areas of practice are chosen, for which standards are designed. It is impossible to carry out an audit unless there is a standard against which practice can be measured.

Step 1: Set the standards

It has been stated above that ideally standards should be incorporated with the CTP and/or the SOPs. Below is an example of standards relating to the recording of treatments.

At the end of the treatment the therapist will have:

- written the date of the assessment in full

- stated the name of the therapy offered

- included a completed assessment form signed by the patient

- included written notes which recorded the treatment given

- signed the notes he/she has written using the signature in the signature bank.

Step 2: Collect data to measure practice

Once the decision has been made to carry out an audit, the standards which are to be measured and by which department must also be agreed. First, the CT lead needs to agree with service managers and the relevant staff that an audit of the complementary therapy notes will be taking place during a certain timescale. He/she needs to identify the number of patients' records suitable for audit and how he/she will gain access to the notes (bearing in mind that they are likely to be used by a multidisciplinary team). Supposing the CT lead decides to audit the previous 20 patients who had an initial treatment prior to the date of the audit, if the five standards above are chosen, this will result in 100 items of data to be collected, analyzed, written up, and the outcomes distributed before action plans are agreed and implemented.

If the complementary therapy notes are kept separately from the main patient's notes they will probably be more easily accessible. However, if therapists write directly on the main paper notes, or in the electronic notes for the patient, access can be more complex and time-consuming. Not every patient will have received complementary therapy and the CT lead may need to go through several sets of notes before those which meet the criteria for audit can be identified.

A method of recording the data needs to be set up and times arranged when access to the notes is available.

The emphasis needs to be on developing the service, rather than therapists feeling that they are being 'examined' or watched. Therapists need to be informed of the process and some of them may be willing to assist. It is suggested that it is better to audit a 'key' area well, rather than trying to do a major audit of the whole service.

Step 3: Collate outcomes and give feedback

Once the data has been collected and analyzed, the outcomes need to be compared with the original standards so the 'gaps' can be identified as well as the areas which are working well.

A report needs to be written for circulation to therapists and managers of services involved. Both groups will need feedback, either separately or together. It is important that the feedback is non-judgmental and anonymous, with any areas requiring further training or adjustments to the processes identified.

Step 4: Reflect and agree action plans

Following the feedback, meetings will need to be arranged where plans are devised in order to address areas where standards are not being met. There may be a need for additional therapist training, developing revised systems and/or liaising with other services. It is important to include realistic targets in terms of time. At this stage, it may also be necessary to consider a revision of the existing standards.

Step 5: Implement revised practices

When implementing a training program and integrating the revised practices with the service, it is important that realistic dates for completion are scheduled. Unless this time allocation is built into the audit system, it is all too easy for the cycle to be broken and the purposes of the audit to be lost.

Step 6: Re-audit

As the process described is a 'cyclical audit,' there needs to be a re-audit of standards at the end of an agreed time period, so the effectiveness of the changes can be assessed.

Although the audit process can be challenging, it does give the CT service a high profile as it portrays a high degree of efficiency and professionalism of service delivery. It turns the documentation into 'real-time relevance' rather than being a 'paper' exercise. The CT lead is able to liaise with healthcare professionals and other members of staff who would not normally come into direct contact with the complementary therapy service. It also enables therapists to be involved in the development and efficiency of the service which they provide, and to offer opportunities for their own professional development.

SUMMARY

This chapter has focused on the importance of the documentation that supports the complementary therapy service. While acknowledging the time involved in writing the initial, documents, it is essential that all CT services have policies and standard operating procedures. Standards are an implicit part of both policies and SOPs as they will enable evaluation through carrying out an audit as per the described process.

REFERENCES

Department of Health (2010) *Essence of Care*. London: DoH.

Fearon, J. (2006) 'Developing a Complementary Therapy Policy.' *British Journal of Nursing 15*, 4, 228–232.

Murphy, H. (2009) 'How audit can improve a service.' *In Essence 8*, 2, 14–18.

Stone, J. (2010) 'Professional, Ethical and Legal Issues in Hypnotherapy.' In A. Cawthorn and. P. Mackereth (eds) *Integrative Hypnotherapy: Complementary Approaches in Clinical Care*. London; Elsevier.

Tavares, M. (2005) *Guide for Writing Policies, Procedures and Protocols: Complementary Therapies in Supportive and Palliative Care*. London: Help the Hospices.

Warren, T., Freer, S., Molinari, M. (2011) 'Developing an end of life benchmark in acute care.' *Nursing Times 107*, 43, 15–17.

Chapter 5

EVALUATING THE EVIDENCE

Graeme Donald and Rebecca Knowles

KEY WORDS
research, methods, randomized controlled
trial, qualitative research, CAM

INTRODUCTION

Complementary therapists may find themselves working in a variety of settings, particularly private practice, hospices, a vast array of charitable organizations and even large hospitals. Depending on the context, an ability to apply research evidence to their practice may be important in the discharge of their roles. Some may even be in a position to consider driving their own research forward.

This chapter provides an overview of the evidence-based paradigm that current healthcare operates within, and acknowledges some issues that are specific to the research of complementary and alternative medicine (CAM) interventions, such as aromatherapy, massage and relaxation. A selection of recent research studies will be presented that include both the innovative application of certain therapies and results that may be of particular interest (see Figure 5.1).

EVIDENCE-BASED PRACTICE AND RESEARCH DESIGNS

Since its development in the 1990s, evidence-based practice (EBP) has become a pivotal component of healthcare delivery. When considered at its most basic, EBP is about driving the application of best practice and best evidence, ensuring the most cost-effective use of resources. When examined more closely, it is, of course, much more complex than this; however, it is not the aim of this chapter to explore this in depth, simply to provide a context. In the case of CAM interventions like massage, aromatherapy and relaxation, the question that arises is what constitutes said evidence.

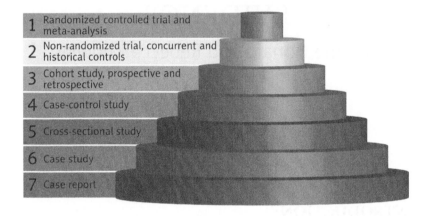

Figure 5.1: Hierarchy of evidence (adapted from Sackett et al. 2000)

With the advent of EBP, a hierarchy of evidence was proposed by Sackett *et al.* (2000), dictating the relative strength of different research designs. The proposition was that any study design which was higher up the hierarchy was considered to be stronger, and at less risk of bias, than those further down the hierarchy. This principle enables the reader to take the findings of the research more seriously. Summaries of the main research methods likely to be encountered are outlined below.

Randomized controlled trial (RCT): A type of experimental scientific study where participants are randomly allocated to one type of treatment or another. Patients in each group follow the same path (for example, tests, procedures, timing) with the only difference being the type of treatment they receive. Controlling external factors and using random allocation leads to lower bias in the study, making the results more reliable. This is considered the gold standard of healthcare research.

Systematic review and meta-analysis: A research study where the academic databases are methodically searched for all relevant papers on a particular subject, for example massage in treating depression in cancer patients. Papers are selected on pre-specified criteria to limit bias during the searching process. Meta-analysis is, when possible, where the results of all papers are analysed to calculate an aggregate, leading to a more categorical conclusion, based on several studies, thus strengthening the results. Often, the results of systematic reviews are based on combining the results of several RCTs, leading to a general acceptance that this kind of (secondary) research sits at the pinnacle of the hierarchy of evidence.

Non-randomized trial: Sometimes called a quasi-experiment, this design is similar to an RCT except that it does not include random allocation. Attempts are still made to control external factors, but patients are allocated to their treatment group using a non-random method such as patient self-selection or alternate allocation.

Cohort study: An observational type of research where a cohort (a group of people who share similar characteristics) are explored for the effects of a particular characteristic or experience, for example people within a given age range who were given a specific vaccination, or people living with cancer who started regular massage sessions early in their journey. Cohort studies are longitudinal i.e. participants are followed over a period of time.

Cross-sectional study: The purpose of this approach is describing the nature and status of a phenomenon of interest, or for describing relationships within that phenomenon at one specific time point. It explores correlation, rather than causation. Surveys and opinion polls are the most common examples of this study design.

Case study: An analysis of a person, group, event and so on, studied via one or more methods. Case studies may include varied data like quantitative, statistical testing or qualitative data generated from patient interviews or responses to questionnaires. There are several formal methodologies proposed for guiding case study research.

Case report: This is a report of a specific patient and their symptoms, diagnosis, treatment and outcomes. Often, case reports highlight unexpected observations or document the effect of new treatments.

Single group pre-post test design: A research design where a group of people are all exposed to a particular treatment. They are evaluated before and after receiving the treatment to investigate any differences.

This method of research is accepted as being subject to bias, given the lack of a comparison group. It is often used in pilot studies to produce evidence of whether or not it is appropriate to expose the treatment in question to further, more expensive, research methods.

Qualitative research: This type of research is particularly interested in the human experience and explores it directly, using methods such as focus groups and interviews. A vital principle in qualitative research is that direct experience is too complex to be reduced to a set of numbers and attempts to represent this using textual and interpretive results drawn from the words of participants. Several rigorous methodologies (such as thematic analysis, grounded theory, phenomenology) can be applied to offset the arguably subjective nature of this kind of research. Furthermore, involving more than one person in analysis also ensures that the results are reliable.

Not all of these research designs are included in the hierarchy of evidence, highlighting its limitations, which have been acknowledged in a range of situations. The RCT has been presented as the gold standard of clinical research its three defining components of control, randomization and manipulation (Polit and Beck 2004) leading to a lowered risk of bias. By attempting to eliminate all other possible factors that may affect the results of the research, any changes in patient outcomes are more likely to have resulted from the intervention under investigation; thus the findings are more reliable. Despite the relative strengths of the RCT, some aspects of EBP and the hierarchy of evidence have come under criticism. Cohen, Stavri and Hersch (2004) seriously questioned the narrow definition of evidence and the lack of focus on the individual. Indeed, Lambert (2006) also identified a lack of engagement with individual patient views. If EBP is about making sure that best practice is promoted then, surely, the opinions and experiences of the recipients of care should be taken into account.

Person-centred care is usually of particular interest to complementary therapists and has been defined as (a) exploring both the disease and the illness experience, (b) understanding the whole person, (c) finding common ground regarding management, (d) incorporating prevention and health promotion and (e) enhancing the practitioner-patient relationship (Little *et al.* 2001; Stewart *et al.* 2003). The inclusion of qualitative research has advanced the development of person-centred care in areas of medicine like stroke, cancer and fertility (Dancet *et al.* 2011; Kvale and Bondevik 2008; Lawrence and Kinn 2011) and is being increasingly used in applied healthcare research. Much qualitative research explores the nature of a person's felt experience, and values the individual focus and the richness of the textual and interpretive data collected. Process evaluations, often involving qualitative methods, focus on questions such as 'how' and 'why' a healthcare intervention works. Such evaluations include elements like participants' views and their experience of the intervention in question (Craig *et al.* 2008; Oakley *et al.* 2006; Pincus *et al.* 2013). This is in line with a campaign for 'real evidence-based medicine', where Greenhalgh, Howick and Maskrey (2014) reiterate the need for focusing on the individual, in addition to producing evidence that is usable and robust. This movement is philosophically aligned with the practitioners of complementary medicine and is a promising avenue when exploring the integration of aromatherapy, massage and relaxation with the mainstream.

CHALLENGES SPECIFIC TO CAM RESEARCH

The RCT and the limitations of its methods have also proven to be contentious in CAM research. This has been debated in the literature and is based on the complexity of CAM practices, like massage or aromatherapy, and on their underlying philosophical principles (Aickin 2010; Fischer *et al.* 2012; Fonnebo *et al.* 2007; House of Lords 2000; Mason, Tovey and Long 2002; Pirotta 2007; Verhoef *et al.* 2005) As part of CAMbrella, (an EU-wide project to develop a roadmap for CAM research) Fischer *et al.* (2012) conducted a systematic review of the methodological issues inherent in CAM research. The reader is encouraged to source this paper and to read it in full.

The belief among many CAM practitioners is that the combined effect of these components is greater than the sum of its parts. It is common in clinical research to isolate and test components of interventions; however, many feel that this is anathema to the spirit of the CAM method, and by dissecting it, the resultant research may lead to an underestimation of effect. One solution to this problem is to research overall effectiveness, or to use refined research methods that can take account of this CAM's complexities.

As a corollary, clinical research values the standardization of treatments so as to ensure validity of the results, and to assure confidence that all research participants experienced exactly the same procedures. While this strategy is useful in evaluating interventions that have been standardized during their development phase (for example health education courses), it poses a problem for researching CAM. Proponents of CAM claim that the individualization of treatments is a unique strength that contributes to the overall treatment effect, thus their argument is that standardizing CAM treatments leads to reduced effect. However, others argue that the individualization of treatment hinders the repeatability of trials, which is a vital principle in the application of the scientific method. Possible solutions to this issue include the use of semi-standardized treatment protocols. This is where a core treatment is provided to all participants, but where the therapist may employ pre-defined adaptations, dependent on the needs assessment of the participant. Another solution would be to employ both individualized and standardized treatment options within a research design, allowing direct comparison during analysis of the results.

The final problem discussed in this chapter is the selection of appropriate control groups. Often, CAM research compares a therapy against standard care only. While this can be useful in proof of principle studies, Ernst and Lee (2008) have argued that this design inevitably leads to a positive result; comparing something vs. nothing will most likely yield a difference. Control conditions in CAM research should therefore be based ideally on providing sham/placebo treatment. Such 'treatments' could also be termed 'mock' treatments, where patients believe that they are receiving the genuine therapy but, in reality, they are not. Attention matching is where the control group receives the same level of attention compared with the treatment group. For example, if those in the treatment group receive a one-hour intervention, weekly for six weeks, then the control group should also receive some kind of intervention for one hour, weekly for six weeks. Such an intervention should be considered benign and unlikely to elicit the response sought from the active treatment.

From their results, Fischer *et al.* (2012) conclude that research methods applicable to conventional medicine should be applied to CAM. RCTs are able to produce viable evidence in this field, but they need to be adapted appropriately to take CAM-specific issues into account. As previously identified, RCTs cannot answer all research questions; however the inclusion of qualitative methods can be used to explore the subjective views of individuals, thus gaining understanding of the person-centred experience of the intervention. The logical conclusion of these arguments is that there is a place for each method in CAM research, depending on the situation and the research questions to be answered. Walach *et al.* (2006) support this position, committing to the principle that the methods of research employed should be driven by the questions being asked, and not by simply following a rigid hierarchy.

It is also worth appreciating that research methods are sometimes constrained by the setting in which they are applied; it may be more practical to evaluate a CAM intervention as it is delivered in practice, without randomization or a control group, because of logistical or ethical concerns. Similarly, for an emerging area of CAM practice, small-scale research investigating proof of principle may be necessary, and justified, before moving on to applying more complex and costly methods.

LITERATURE REVIEWING AND CRITICAL APPRAISAL

Identifying and evaluating the evidence that underpins massage, aromatherapy and relaxation is of paramount importance in guiding a therapist's practice. For example, there may be situations where a therapy, like aromatherapy, has been shown to not be effective. Therapists may react in one of three ways to this – phasing out this approach from their existing practice, responsively adapting their practice, or retaining a belief that it works, and carrying on regardless despite the research evidence. The third option is not advised: doing so would violate the philosophy of EBP and present serious ethical concerns about working in the patient's best interests.

ACCESSING PAPERS

The first problem is how to find and obtain access to available research papers. Therapists working within academic or clinical settings may have access to the established academic databases, like MEDLINE, through which they will be able to find relevant papers. This will be dependent on their institution's subscription. Failing this, papers may be found through local libraries or by searching through Google Scholar. Although not generally accepted as a rigorous method of searching the literature, a therapist with no other access may find this function useful. Often, whole papers can be viewed and downloaded using Google Scholar.

For conducting formal literature reviews that attempt to identify all papers in a given context, there are entire books providing guidance on the methods used. Anyone attempting a comprehensive literature search should seek such guidance.

CRITICAL APPRAISAL

When reading and absorbing the research evidence, it is important to be able to apply a critical eye to the methods used by the researchers, so that the results are not simply unquestioningly accepted. When evaluating quantitative research, like RCTs, particular concerns arise in the power of the statistical testing used. The accuracy is improved with higher numbers of research participants, and also in the methods used to control potential bias. These methods include random allocation and concealing the allocation from all members of the team. If team members are aware of the allocation, they may behave differently toward the participant and elicit a false positive, known as the placebo effect. Similarly, to avoid elicitation of the placebo effect, the allocation may be concealed from the participants themselves. The level of participant attrition in a trial may also affect the reliability of the results and needs to be taken into consideration. A data analysis strategy called Intention to Treat (ITT) analysis is often employed to manage the bias introduced by participants pulling out of the research. There are different methods of doing this, but they all include making sure that missing data is replaced by a statistical estimate that enables participants' data to still be included in the analysis.

A checklist for evaluating a report of a non-pharmacological trial (CLEAR NPT) is presented in Table 5.1 (Boutron *et al.* 2005). This is a quality appraisal tool that can help you to critique research; it is suitable for applying to any trial that is not assessing the effectiveness of a new drug. Attention should be paid to the issue of blinding. The advantage of CLEAR NPT is that it takes into account that blinding may be impossible in evaluating some non-pharmaceutical interventions. For example, when comparing surgery to taking medication, both the surgeon and the patient are aware of whether or not the patient has received surgery or the medication. Similarly, participants may well be aware that they are receiving a massage or having a relaxation script delivered to them.

In appraising the quality of qualitative research, other tools – that are fit for purpose – are available. The tool proposed by the UK Critical Appraisal Skills Programme (CASP) is commonly used and includes questions focusing on the appropriateness of the methods used and the transparency and rigor of data analysis techniques used.

Table 5.1: Checklist for evaluating a report of a non-pharmacological trial (CLEAR NPT)

1. Was the generation of allocation sequences adequate?	Yes	
	No	
	Unclear	
2. Was the treatment allocation concealed?	Yes	
	No	
	Unclear	
3. Were details of the intervention administered to each group made available?	Yes	
	No	
	Unclear	
4. Were care providers' experience or skill in each arm appropriate?	Yes	
	No	
	Unclear	
5. Was participant (i.e. patients) adherence assessed quantitatively?	Yes	
	No	
	Unclear	
6. Were participants adequately blinded?	Yes	
	No (blinding not feasible)	
	No (blinding is feasible)	
	Unclear	
6.1. If participants were not adequately blinded		
6.1.1. Were all other treatments and care (i.e. co-interventions) the same in each randomized group?	Yes	
	No	
	Unclear	
6.1.2. Were withdrawals and lost-to-follow-up the same in each randomized group?	Yes	
	No	
	Unclear	
7. Were care providers or persons caring for the participants adequately blinded?	Yes	
	No (blinding not feasible)	
	No (blinding is feasible)	
	Unclear	

7.1. If care providers were not adequately blinded		
7.1.1. Were all other treatments and care (i.e. cointerventions) the same in each randomized group?	Yes	
	No	
	Unclear	
7.1.2. Were withdrawals and lost-to-follow-up the same in each randomized group?	Yes	
	No	
	Unclear	
8. Were outcome assessors adequately blinded to assess the primary outcomes?	Yes	
	No (blinding not feasible)	
	No (blinding is feasible)	
	Unclear	
8.1. If outcome assessors were not adequately blinded, were specific methods used to avoid ascertainment bias (systematic differences in outcome assessment)?	Yes	
	No	
	Unclear	
9. Was the follow-up schedule the same in each group?	Yes	
	No	
	Unclear	
10. Were the main outcomes analyzed according to the intention-to-treat principle?	Yes	
	No	
	Unclear	

(Boutron *et al.* 2005)

SUMMARY

This chapter has provided a general overview of some of the areas of vital importance when considering how to apply research evidence to the practice of complementary therapies such as aromatherapy, massage and relaxation. A range of recent research studies has been offered for consideration but, more importantly, in an attempt to pique your interest and to inspire the spirit of inquiry. Many CAM practitioners are passionate about the work that they do and believe in the therapies that they practise. If this passion and belief is to be harnessed properly, in order to best serve the needs of people, then complementary therapists should be confident in applying rigorous research methods to their practice, so equipping themselves with the knowledge and ability to thoughtfully and critically apply the latest research. (Tables of research follow and references are at the end.)

Table 5.2: Selected massage research 2008–13

Study	Objective	Design	Outcome measures	Results	Comments
Stringer, Swindell and Dennis (2008)	To identify whether single 20-minute massage sessions were safe and effective in reducing stress levels of isolated haematological oncology patients.	A pilot study based on a randomized controlled trial; patients were randomized to aromatherapy, massage or a rest (control) arm (n=39).	Primary outcome measure was the fall in serum cortisol levels and prolactin levels. Semi-structured interviews. Quality of life questionnaire (EORTC QLQ-C30).	A significant difference was seen between arms in cortisol (p=0.002) and prolactin (p=0.031) levels from baseline to 30 minutes post-session. Aromatherapy and massage arms showed a significantly greater drop in cortisol than the rest arm. Only the massage arm had a significantly greater reduction in prolactin than the rest arm. The questionnaires showed a significant reduction in 'need for rest' for patients in both experimental arms compared with the control arm. The interviews identified a universal feeling of relaxation in patients in the experimental arms.	This study demonstrated that in isolated haematological oncology patients, a significant reduction in cortisol could be safely achieved through massage, with associated improvement in psychological wellbeing.
Cronfalk *et al.* (2009)	To explore how patients with cancer in palliative home care experienced soft tissue massage.	Patients received soft tissue massage (hand or foot) nine times over a period of two weeks. Each session lasted 25 minutes. An interview was conducted following the last massage session (n=22).	Qualitative interview.	Soft tissue massage generated feelings of existential respite with perceptions of being released from illness for a while. Two categories constituted the basis of the experiences: 1) 'an experience of thoughtful attention' and 2) 'a sensation of complete tranquility' resulting in the overarching theme 'a time of existential respite'.	The patients experienced the massage as giving meaning and being important as it generated feelings of an inner respite. Soft tissue massage appears to be an appreciated source of support to dying patients in palliative home care.

cont.

Study	Objective	Design	Outcome measures	Results	Comments
Listing *et al.* (2010)	To investigate the efficacy of classical massage on stress perception and mood disturbances in women diagnosed with primary breast cancer.	Patients were randomized to an intervention or control group. For a period of five weeks the intervention group received biweekly 30-minute classical massages. The control group received no additional treatment to their routine healthcare. Patients' blood was collected at baseline (T1), at the end of the intervention period (T2), and six weeks after T2 (T3) (n=34).	Perceived stress questionnaire. Berlin mood questionnaire. Blood results.	Compared with the control group, women in the intervention group reported significantly lower mood disturbances, especially for anger (p=0.048), anxious depression (p=0.03) at T2, and tiredness at T3 (p=0.01). Perceived stress and cortisol serum levels (p=0.03) were significantly reduced after massage therapy (T2) compared with baseline in the intervention group.	The study suggests that women with breast cancer benefited from a five-week massage treatment. The study suggests that massage therapy may lead to a short-term reduction of stress perception and cortisol levels. Furthermore, here was a positive impact of massage on mood disturbances.
Toth *et al.* (2013)	To determine the feasibility and effects of providing therapeutic massage at home for patients with metastatic cancer.	Randomized controlled trial. Patients were allocated to one of three groups: <ul><li>massage therapy (intervention)</li><li>no-touch intervention (control)</li><li>usual care (control).</li></ul> Massage therapy was provided in patients' homes. They received up to three treatments, lasting between 15 and 45 minutes. For the no-touch intervention the therapist held his/her hands 12 inches over the patient's body (n=42).	Primary: pain, anxiety and alertness. Secondary: quality of life and sleep.	A significant improvement was found in the quality of life of the patients who received massage therapy after one-week follow-up, which was not observed in either of the control groups, but the difference was not sustained at one month. There were trends towards improvement in pain and sleep of the patients after therapeutic massage but not in patients in the control groups.	Providing therapeutic massage improves the quality of life at the end of life for patients and may be associated with further beneficial effects, such as improvement in pain and sleep quality.

| Kutner *et al.* (2008) | To evaluate the efficacy of massage for decreasing pain and symptom distress and improving quality of life among persons with advanced cancer. | Multi-site, prospective, two-group, randomized, single-blind trial.

Six 30-minute massage or simple touch sessions over two weeks for patients with moderate to severe pain. Simple touch consisted of placing both hands on the patients for three minutes at various locations (n=380). | Primary: immediate and sustained change in pain.

Secondary: immediate change in mood and 60-second heart and respiratory rates.

Sustained change in quality of life. Symptom distress and analgesic medication use. | Both groups demonstrated immediate improvement in pain and mood.

Massage was superior for both immediate pain and mood (p<0.001).

No between-group mean differences occurred over time in sustained pain, quality of life, symptom distress or analgesic medication use. | Massage may have immediately beneficial effects on pain and mood among patients with advanced cancer.

Given the lack of sustained effects and the observed improvements in both study groups, the potential benefits of attention and simple touch should also be considered in this patient population. |

Table 5.3: Selected aromatherapy research 2009–14

Study	Objective	Design	Outcome measures	Results	Comments
Stringer and Donald (2011)	To evaluate the effects of a new aromatherapy intervention introduced within an acute cancer care setting in the UK.	A retrospective service evaluation. Patients referred to the complementary therapy service were, if appropriate, offered an aromastick. If the offer was accepted, patients' details were captured on an evaluation form. One week later the patients were followed up by a different therapist (n=160).	Frequency of using the aromastick and perceived benefits.	77% of all patients reported deriving at least one benefit from the aromastick. In anxious patients, 65% reported feeling more relaxed and 51% felt less stress. 47% of nauseous patients said that the aromastick had settled their nausea and 55% of those experiencing sleep disturbances felt that the aromastick helped them sleep.	The results suggest that the effects of the aromastick may be directly proportional to the frequency of their use. The data presented in this paper highlights the potential for aromasticks within the clinical setting.
Dyer et al. (2014)	To consider the use of aromasticks in a cancer centre in the UK.	A retrospective clinical audit covering a 28-month period, reporting on current clinical practice. Patients that were seen by the complementary therapy team at the centre either requested or were offered an aromastick. Essential oils for the aromasticks were chosen by the patients themselves in conjunction with the therapist. Aromastick use was documented, data from which was collected and reviewed (n=514).	Documentation of aromastick use.	Patient compliance was high and there were no reported ill effects. A blend of lavender and eucalyptus was 'hugely successful' in alleviating nausea, encouraging deep breathing and increasing relaxation. There was positive feedback in the use of citrus oils for increasing appetite and encouraging patients to eat, and providing relief to patients who were unable to eat but missed the sensations of eating.	Aromasticks can be individualized to suit each patient's needs and preferences. Blends of oils can be used to minimize the chance of negative odour associations to familiar odours, particularly in situations with a negative emotional context, such as chemotherapy-induced nausea and vomiting. Patients can use blends they have enjoyed (positive odour association). Informal feedback from patients demonstrates the popularity and perceived effectiveness of aromasticks for a wide range of symptoms. Aromasticks continue to be a useful, simple, popular and cost-effective addition to the ways in which patients can be treated.

| Maddocks-Jennings et al. (2009) | To evaluate the effects of a mouthwash containing the essential oils Leptospermum scoparium (manuka) and Kunzea ericoides (kanuka) on radiation-induced mucositis of the oropharyngeal area during treatment for head and neck cancers. | A randomized, placebo-controlled feasibility study with a convenience sample. Patients were sequentially allocated to an active gargle (one drop of each essential oil), placebo gargle (sterile water) or control group. Gargling commenced up to two days before radiotherapy and continued for one week. Patients gargled three to five times per day for at least 15 seconds; 30 minutes before or after eating, smoking or drinking, as well as before and after radiotherapy. Patients completed a daily diary recording their pain scores, medication use and other oral symptoms. At a weekly clinical review, oral mucosa was graded and body weight and general wellbeing were recorded. Patients were followed up for at least two weeks and completed a survey recording the severity of oral symptoms at each stage of treatment (n=19). | The development of mucositis (Modified Radiation Therapy Oncology Group Scale of Acute Toxicities). Pain (visual analogue scale). Nutritional effects (weekly weight change, taste, appetite, ability to eat, dry mouth, nausea, vomiting and day-to-day functioning). | Those in the essential oil group were observed to have a delayed onset of mucositis, reduced pain and oral mucositis symptoms relative to the placebo and the control groups. In addition, those in the essential oil group were seen to have less weight loss (1%) than the other two groups (control 2.5%, placebo 4.5%). | The results support the hypothesis that very small volumes of manuka and kanuka used in a gargle can provide a positive effect on the development of radiation-induced mucositis. This has been shown to be a simple, effective, cost-effective, easy-to-administer and novel treatment for what is recognized as a cause of significant discomfort and pain in those undergoing radiotherapy for head and neck cancer, and for which there is currently no definitive treatment. |

Table 5.4: Selected relaxation research 2008–11

Study	Objective	Design	Outcome measures	Results	Comments
Kwekkeboom, Abbott-Anderson and Wanta (2010)	To evaluate the feasibility of a patient-controlled cognitive behavioural intervention for pain, fatigue and sleep disturbance during advanced cancer, and to assess initial efficacy of the intervention in controlling symptoms.	One-group pre-test-post-test design in adults with advanced colorectal, lung, prostate or gynaecologic cancer receiving chemotherapy or radiotherapy at outpatient oncology clinics in a comprehensive cancer centre. Patients completed baseline measures and received training to use an MP3 player loaded with 12 cognitive-behavioural strategies (relaxation exercises, guided imagery, and nature sound recordings). Patients used these as needed for symptom management, keeping a log of symptom ratings with each use. Following the two-week intervention, patients completed a second symptom inventory and an evaluation of the intervention (n=30).	Feasibility. Patient-controlled cognitive behavioural intervention. Pain. Fatigue. Sleep disturbance.	The majority of participants reported that they enjoyed the intervention, had learned useful skills and perceived improvement in their symptoms. Symptom scores at two weeks did not differ significantly from baseline; however, significant reductions in pain, fatigue and sleep disturbance severity were found in ratings made immediately before and after the use of a cognitive behavioural strategy.	The patient-controlled cognitive behavioural intervention could reduce day-to-day severity of co-occurring pain, fatigue and sleep disturbance.
Fenlon, Corner and Haviland (2008)	To assess the efficacy of relaxation training in reducing the incidence of hot flashes in women with primary breast cancer.	Randomized controlled trial. The intervention group received a single, hour-long, one-to-one relaxation training session, which included the basics of stress management, written information, breathing techniques, muscle relaxation and guided imagery. An audio tape of the trainer's voice talking through the same relaxation session was given to the women to use at home for 20 minutes each day for at least a month. All measures were completed at baseline, and one and three months after relaxation training (n=150).	Incidence of flashes (diary). Severity of flashes (pre-defined categories based on work by Finck et al.). Distress caused by flashes (Hunter menopause scale). Quality of life (functional assessment of cancer therapy and endocrine subscale). Anxiety (Spielberger State/Trait Anxiety Index).	The incidence and severity of hot flashes each significantly declined over one month (p<0.001 and p=0.01 respectively), compared with the control group. Distress caused by flashes also significantly declined in the treatment group over one month (p=0.01), compared with the control group.	There may be real benefits for some women who use relaxation for the relief of hot flashes. Relaxation may be a useful component of a programme of measures to relieve hot flashes in women with primary breast cancer.

REFERENCES

Aickin, M. (2010) 'Comparative effectiveness research and CAM.' *Journal of Alternative and Complementary Medicine 16,* 1, 1–2.

Boutron, I., Moher, D., Tugwell, P., Giraudeau, B. *et al.* (2005) 'A checklist to evaluate a report of a non-pharmacological trial (CLEAR NPT) was developed using consensus.' *Journal of Clinical Epidemiology 58,* 12, 1233–1240.

Cohen, A., Stavri, P., Hersch, W. (2004) 'A categorisation and analysis of the criticisms of evidence-based medicine.' *International Journal of Medical Informatics, 73,* 1, 35–43.

Craig, P., Dieppe, P., MacIntyre, S., Michie, S., Nazereth, I., Pettigrew, M. (2008) 'Developing and evaluating complex interventions: the new Medical Research Council guidance.' *British Medical Journal 337,* 7676, 979–983.

Critical Appraisal Skills Programme (CASP). Available at www.casp-uk.net, accessed on 1 December 2015.

Cronfalk, B.S., Strang, P., Ternestedt, B.M., Friedrichsen, M. (2009) 'The existential experiences of receiving soft tissue massage in palliative home care—an intervention.' *Supportive Care in Cancer 1,* 9, 1203–1211.

Dancet, E., Van Empel, I., Rober, P., Nelen, W., Kremer, J., D'Hooghe, T. (2011) 'Patient-centred infertility care: a qualitative study to listen to the patient's voice.' *Human Reproduction 26,* 4, 827–833.

Dyer, J., Cleary, L., Ragsdale-Lowe, M., McNeill, S., Osland, C. (2014) 'The use of aromasticks at a cancer centre: A retrospective audit.' *Complementary Therapies in Clinical Practice 20,* 4, 203–206.

Ernst, E. and Lee, M. (2008) 'A trial design that generates only "positive" results.' *Journal of Postgraduate Medicine 54,* 3, 214–216.

Fenlon, D.R., Corner, J.L., Haviland, J.S. (2008) 'A randomized controlled trial of relaxation training to reduce hot flashes in women with primary breast cancer.' *Journal of Pain and Symptom Management 35,* 4, 397–405.

Fischer, H.F., Junne, F., Witt, C., von Ammon, K., Cardini, F., Fonnebo, V. (2012) 'Key issues in clinical and epidemiological research in CAM: a systematic literature review.' *Forschende Komplementmed 19,* 9 (suppl. 2) 51–60.

Fonnebo, V., Grimsgaard, S., Walach, H., Ritenbaugh C. *et al.* (2007) 'Researching complementary and alternative treatments – the gatekeepers are not at home.' *BMC Medical Research Methodology 7.* DOI: 10.1186/1471-2288-7-7.

Greenhalgh, T. Howick, J., Maskrey, N. (2014) 'Evidence-based medicine: a movement in crisis?' *British Medical Journal,* 2014: 348.

House of Lords Select Committee on Science and Technology (2000) *Complementary and Alternative Medicine.* London: The Stationery Office.

Kutner, J.S., Smith, M.C., Corbin, L., Hemphill, L. *et al.* (2008) 'Massage therapy versus simple touch to improve pain and mood in patients with advanced cancer: a randomized trial.' *Annals of Internal Medicine 149,* 6, 369–379.

Kvale, K. and Bondevik, M. (2008) 'What is important for patient-centred care? A qualitative study about the perceptions of patients with cancer.' *Scandinavian Journal of Caring Sciences 22,* 4, 582–589.

Kwekkeboom, K.L., Abbott-Anderson, K., Wanta, B. (2010) 'Feasibility of a patient-controlled cognitive behavioral intervention for pain, fatigue, and sleep disturbance in cancer.' *Oncology Nursing Forum 37,* 3, E151. NIH Public Access.

Lambert, H. (2006) 'Accounting for EBM: notions of evidence in medicine.' *Social Science and Medicine, 62,* 11, 2633–2645.

Lawrence, M. and Kinn, S. (2011) 'Defining and measuring patient-centred care: an example from a mixed methods systematic review of the stroke literature.' *Health Expectations 15*, 3, 295–326.

Listing, M., Krohn, M., Liezmann, C., Kim, I. *et al.* (2010) 'The efficacy of classical massage on stress perception and cortisol following primary treatment of breast cancer.' *Archives of Women's Mental Health 13*, 2, 165–173.

Little, P., Everitt, H., Williamson, I., Warner, G. *et al.* (2001) 'Preferences of patients for patient-centred approach to consultation in primary care: an observational study.' *British Medical Journal 323*, 7284, 1–7.

Maddocks-Jennings, W., Wilkinson, J. M., Cavanagh, H.M., Shillington, D. (2009) 'Evaluating the effects of the essential oils leptospermum scoparium (manuka) and kunzea ericoides (kanuka) on radiotherapy induced mucositis: a randomized, placebo controlled feasibility study.' *European Journal of Oncology Nursing 13*, 2, 87–93.

Mason, S., Tovey, P., Long, A. (2002) 'Evaluating complementary medicine: methodological challenges of randomized controlled trials.' *British Medical Journal* 325, 7368, 832–834.

Oakley, A., Strange, V., Bonell, C., Allen, E., Stephenson, J. (2006) 'Process evaluation in randomized controlled trials of complex interventions.' *British Medical Journal 332*, 7538, 413–416.

Pincus, T., Anwar, S., McCracken, L., McGregor, A. *et al.* (2013) 'Testing the credibility, feasibility and acceptability of an optimised behavioural intervention (OBI) for avoidant low back pain patients: protocol for a ranodomized feasibility study.' *Trials 14*. DOI: 10.1186/1745-6215-14-172

Polit, D.F. and Beck, C.T. (2004) *Nursing Research: Principles and Methods.* Philadelphia. Lippincott, Williams and Wilkins.

Pirotta, M. (2007) 'Towards the Application of RCTs for CAM: Methodological Challenges.' In J. Adams (ed.) *Researching Complementary and Alternative Medicine.* London: Routledge.

Sackett, D.L., Straus, S.E., Richardson, W. C., Rosenberg, W., Haynes, B. (2000) *Evidence-based Medicine: How to Practice and Teach EBM.* New York: Churchill Livingstone.

Stewart, M., Brown, J., Weston, W., McWhinney, I. *et al.* (2003) *Patient-centred Medicine: Transforming the Clinical Method.* Abingdon: Radcliffe Medical Press.

Stringer, J. and Donald, G. (2011) 'Aromasticks in cancer care: an innovation not to be sniffed at.' *Complementary Therapies in Clinical Practice 17*, 2, 116–121.

Stringer, J., Swindell, R., Dennis, M. (2008) 'Massage in patients undergoing intensive chemotherapy reduces serum cortisol and prolactin.' *Psycho-Oncology 17*, 10, 1024–1031.

Toth, M., Marcantonio, E.R., Davis, R.B., Walton, T., Kahn, J.R., Phillips, R.S. (2013) 'Massage therapy for patients with metastatic cancer: a pilot randomized controlled trial.' *The Journal of Alternative and Complementary Medicine 19*, 7, 650–656.

Verhoef, M., Lewith, G., Ritenbaugh, C., Boon, H., Fleishman, S., Leis, A. (2005) 'Complementary and alternative medicine whole systems research: beyond identification of the inadequacies of the RCT.' *Complementary Therapies in Medicine 13*, 3, 206–212.

Walach, H., Falkenberg, T., Fonnebo, V., Lewith, G., Jonas, W. (2006) 'Circular instead of hierarchical: methodological principles for the evaluation of complex interventions.' *BMC Medical Research Methodology 6*. DOI: 10.1186/1471-2288-6-29

Chapter 6

EMBEDDING A PALLIATIVE CARE THERAPY SERVICE

Dr Peter A. Mackereth, Paula Maycock, Anita Mehrez and Lydia Nightingale

KEY WORDS
palliative, supportive, service review, specialist therapists

INTRODUCTION

This chapter reports on a service review of a bespoke palliative care complementary therapy service over its first three years. Over 2870 treatment sessions were provided to patients referred directly by the palliative care team, often with complex concerns and issues. Seventy-two per cent were female, with gynaecological, gastro-intestinal, breast and lung cancers forming the largest diagnostic groups. Typical post-treatment comments included: 'soothing', 'calming,' 'bliss' and 'pain eased'. Examples of three composite case studies and recommendations for developing a specialist complementary therapy service in palliative care are given. The purpose of this chapter is to share our service review process and the findings and to make recommendations for this activity.

BACKGROUND

Internationally, there is evidence that complementary therapies are increasingly being provided within cancer and palliative care services, with the development of bespoke and skilled teams of therapists (Andrews and Mackereth 2012; Nyatanga 2015; Vandergrift 2013). Following a review of a cancer hospital service at a north-west UK centre, the complementary therapy team identified the need to improve the frequency of sessions and the range of interventions for palliative care and end-of-life referrals. In 2011, two specialist palliative care (SPC) therapists were appointed to develop both in- and outpatient services; their combined skills included massage, HEARTS, reflexology, aromatherapy, acupuncture and hypnotherapy. The SPC therapists attend multidisciplinary team meetings and case reviews, which include medical staff, clinical nurse specialists, occupational therapists, physiotherapists and the chaplaincy team.

The SPC therapists also provide information to patients and their families about complementary therapy and cancer care services in their own localities. Aside from providing services, the therapists have also been able to contribute towards teaching, research and publication work. Initial project funding permitted attendance at palliative care conferences and study days, with the SPC therapists sharing their learning with the wider complementary therapy team. Additionally, ward-based therapists prioritized palliative care referrals daily, with supervision and support from the SPC therapists. At the time of review, the service was entirely funded from charitable sources, with the majority of interventions carried out in the hospital's wards and outpatient clinics.

Importantly, end-of-life care is complex and challenging. The patient needs to be at the centre of our care, remembering that carers will probably be keeping a vigil at the bedside, hardly stepping out of the room for breaks (see Chapter 14). Nurses and other clinical staff will, no doubt, be respectfully and sensitively checking in with the family and patient, providing essential care. Outside the room, carers might be asked if they need any drinks, extra chairs, information or a complementary therapy either in the room or nearby. SPC therapists have the potential to contribute towards care; sometimes this can be just by being with and listening to patients, carers and staff.

Service evaluations and reviews are a set of procedures to judge the merits of a service by systematic assessment of its aims, objectives, activities, output, outcomes and costs. Anonymized data can be gathered from a variety of sources, but usually includes service users, referrers and the providers. In presenting a report, costs would be itemized as well as other aspects of the provision, such as accommodation, support services, equipment and infrastructure (Gerrish and Mawson 2005). Data can be both retrospective and current in terms of asking service users about their experiences, and referrers about their expectations. Unlike research (see Chapter 5) this activity does not include randomization or control groups, services being delivered as normal. Discussion needs to take place with the relevant research and development (R&D) and audit departments to ascertain whether full ethical approval needs to be sought. It is essential that ethical principles, which are applied to any research and data collection, need to be maintained throughout service evaluations and reviews (Department of Health 2005).

THERAPISTS' SKILLS, KNOWLEDGE AND ROLES
Therapists' skills/knowledge

- ability to work autonomously

- skills in adapting a range of therapies – massage, reflexology, hypnotherapy, stress management techniques, aromatherapy and acupuncture

- commitment to clinical supervision and reflective practice

- ability to teach and support visiting students and new therapists

- knowledge of safeguarding, end-of-life and palliative care issues and principles

- confidence in supporting, directing and referring patients with existential and practical concerns, for example suicidal ideation, spiritual and religious guidance/needs, wills and bereavement support

- knowledge of bereavement and loss theories and concerns.

Roles

- attend weekly palliative care (PC) triage meetings

- maintain referral list – reviewing priorities and frequency of treatment

- assess palliative care referrals

- provide specialist interventions

- support/provide interventions to carers

- work closely with multidisciplinary team members, for example pain services, PC nurses, doctors, chaplaincy

- participate in case reviews

- provide feedback from patients and carers about concerns and issues with the wider multidisciplinary team

- liaise with the psycho-oncology team

- document all treatments

- contribute to the ongoing evaluation and audit activities.

DATA FROM THE SPECIALIST PALLIATIVE CARE COMPLEMENTARY THERAPY SERVICE

All treatments are recorded, with annual data collated and utilized within reports; these are then used in support of internal business cases to the trust's charity board and as evidence of activity and evaluation to external funding bodies. Information gathered via treatment record sheets includes diagnosis, gender, and patient concerns, the interventions provided and post-treatment feedback. In report writing, any data is anonymized. It needs to be acknowledged that patients may give 'positive post-treatment feedback' to please the therapist. Anonymous feedback is helpful both for reflection and making adjustments to future interventions and how services are delivered. Collating themes that reoccur within the data is helpful, not only in exploring therapeutic outcomes for single and combination interventions, but also in providing useful 'soundbites' for report writing and presentations. The data presented here is retrospective; it did not go beyond the analysis of treatment documentation and utilizing an Excel database to generate tables and figures to populate the report.

FINDINGS
The number of patients referred to the service
The Palliative Care Project has enabled the team to deliver over 2870 complementary therapy treatments to patients between

2012 and 2014. Additionally, the wider service has provided support to carers, although whether their loved one was a palliative care referral is not routinely recorded. Since the Palliative Care Project started, the number of patients seen has increased each year (see Figure 6.1). In 2014, 993 palliative care patients were seen; this equated to 8 per cent of the total number of patient sessions provided across the wider hospital (n=12,158).

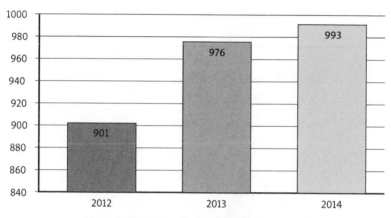

Figure 6.1: Number of palliative care patients seen by the complementary therapy team per year 2012–14

The gender of patients referred and their diagnoses

Figure 6.2 shows that the number of females treated was 2064 (72%) while for males it was 804 (28%). This is due to two reasons:

- The largest diagnostic group for palliative care was gastro-intestinal (n=592) closely followed by gynaecological (n=557) (predominately ovarian cancers) and the third largest group was breast cancer. (See Figure 6.3.)

- There were fewer men referred/requesting complementary therapy support, which appears to be standard throughout the wider hospital service, the ratio being 69 per cent female to 31 per cent male.

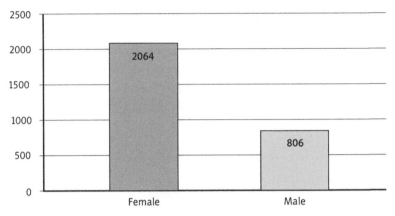

*Figure 6.2: Gender of palliative care patients receiving
a complementary therapy treatment 2012–14*

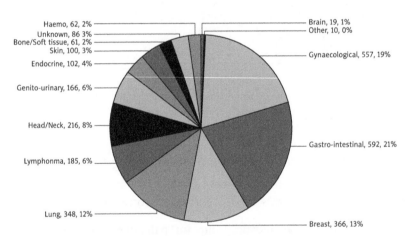

*Figure 6.3: Diagnoses of palliative care patients receiving
a complementary therapy treatment 2012–14*

Patients' concerns

Figure 6.4 shows that there is a cluster of symptoms for which patients are routinely referred to the specialist therapists; these include pain, fatigue, anxiety and worry (n=2870). Throughout the wider hospital complementary therapy service, the standard concerns are anxiety, fatigue and stress. Figure 6.4 demonstrates that palliative care patients report pain as their most significant symptom.

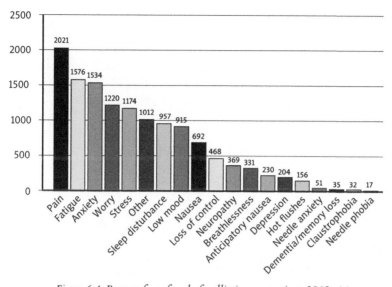

Figure 6.4: Reasons for referral of palliative care patients 2012–14

Treatments received

As the specialist therapists are skilled in a variety of complementary therapies they were able to provide choices to patients with palliative and end-of-life care needs. In line with other services, gentle massage was the most popular; the therapists also provide other interventions, such as stress management techniques, acupuncture, hypnotherapy/ visualization and HEARTS (see Figure 6.5). Table 6.1 details the responses.

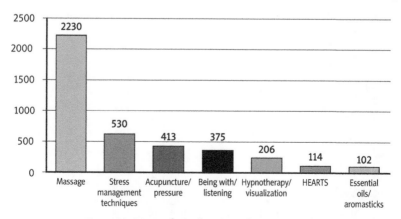

*Figure 6.5: Types of complementary therapy treatments
received by palliative care patients 2012–14*

Table 6.1: Comments made by palliative care patients after receiving a complementary therapy treatment (n=2870)

Categories of comments	Acupuncture n=413	Being with/ listened to n=375	Essential oils/ aromasticks n=102	Hypnotherapy/ visualization n=206	Massage n=2230	Stress management techniques n=630	HEARTS n = 114
Loved/enjoyed	6%	6%	22%	31%	39%	16%	34%
Appreciated	3%	33%	16%	9%	22%	44%	15%
Soothing/calming/relaxing	7%	0%	34%	13%	29%	7%	27%
Helpful	22%	33%	6%	11%	4%	17%	1%
Non-specific comment e.g. information received	13%	22%	6%	6%	1%	10%	10%
Concern or symptom had improved	32%	6%	9%	13%	2%	5%	6%
Pain reduced/gone	8%	0%	6%	17%	2%	1%	4%
Mobility improved	9%	0%	0%	0%	0%	0%	1%

THE SERVICE REVIEW

There were numerous physical symptoms reported, the most common being pain and fatigue. Many were part of a cluster of symptoms linked to treatment side-effects and and/or disease progression. One of the most frequent comments provided by patients after a treatment was 'pain gone' or 'pain reduced'. The data suggests this was most commonly stated comment following acupuncture and hypnotherapy; pain relief was also reported after massage alone in many cases (see Table 6.1, and comments and case study below). As patients present with clusters of symptoms, asking those at the end of life to rate a single symptom before and after treatment would be a burden for them. On another level, outcomes from a complementary therapy session may be different from what was expected or hoped for. The post-treatment comments suggest a level of surprise and gratitude.

Examples of post-treatment comments include:

'You've helped me immeasurably.'

'Really making a huge difference.'

'Can't believe it – life changing.'

'Complementary therapies has given me my life back.'

'Amazed at results.'

'I feel great now!'

'Blissful, thank you.'

'That was beautiful.'

'Absolute joy.'

'It's like being in wonderland.'

'Gorgeous, very special.'

'Better than morphine.'

'Stopped vomiting.'

'Very relaxed and very refreshed.'

'Would have liked it to continue all day.'

'At my wits' end until now.'

Case study 6.1: Easing the pain

Mandy was referred by the Supportive and Palliative Care Team with complex symptoms and was very frail. Due to pain, extensive edema, drains and a catheter, it was difficult for her to find a comfortable position. Her other concerns were anxiety, worry, fatigue, sleeping difficulties and low mood.

After an explanation of the various interventions offered, Mandy requested HEARTS. Initially, the most comfortable position for Mandy was for her to sit at the edge of the bed. First, she received very gentle, slow strokes and light holding over the back and arms. However, this position was not sustainable for Mandy and the therapist suggested re-positioning Mandy's upper body, so that she was leaning over pillows placed on top of the table in front of her. Next, the therapist paid attention to her shoulders, neck and occiput, during which Mandy fell asleep. After ten minutes, Mandy was awake and said, '...that was amazing. I didn't know I could feel like that...what a lovely comfortable position.' Although her condition deteriorated, Mandy was able to continue receiving HEARTS sessions during her four-week stay and went home for end-of-life care, as she wished.

While massage was the most popular intervention, patients often received more than one intervention. Therapists in cancer care are known to offer a 'toolbox' approach, often combining touch with stress management techniques (McLaren *et al.* 2014). These techniques can include guided imagery, hypnotherapy and aromatherapy, the latter in the form of aromasticks (see Chapter 8). The service also includes acupuncture and acupressure, and there is published research about the benefits and experience of receiving these interventions (Mackereth *et al.* 2014; Molassiotis *et al.* 2012).

Massage is acknowledged as offering more than symptom relief in palliative care. Following interviews with 22 patients who had received massage, Cronfalk, Ternestedt and Strang (2009) reported that the patients had perceived it as 'thoughtful attention', 'sensations of tranquility' and 'a time of existential respite'. Beck, Runeson and Blomqvist (2009) have reported that a patient found an 'inner peace' from receiving reported very soft and gentle massage. Comments collated in our review included 'feeling soothed', 'calming' and even 'blissful' (see above and Table 6.1). Stress management and breathing techniques were commonly reported as included in the sessions to equip patients in managing anxiety and distress outside a therapy session (see Chapter 13). Short sessions of hypnotherapy and/or guided imagery (n=206), and aromatherapy (n=102), most frequently provided as an aromastick, were commonly used (see Chapters 8 and 11).

Case study 6.2: A time of bliss

Elizabeth was currently experiencing unremitting nausea and vomiting, pain, anxiety, stress, fatigue and low mood. She had a vomit bowl and a packet of tissues resting on her abdomen. She chose foot massage, selected a preferred aromastick from a choice of three blends and asked for the curtains to be drawn around the bed. Supported into a comfortable position, she was then covered in a soft, warm blanket and encouraged to gently inhale the aromastick, during the oiled foot and lower leg massage. The emphasis was on slow, downward strokes and holding. She closed her eyes, her facial muscles relaxed, breathing deepened and within ten minutes she had drifted into sleep. Feedback on the following day's visit was, 'I remembered my tube (aromastick) and then I went into a blissful dream.'

In our survey, 382 sessions were reported as 'being with', listening, providing information and simple advice, rather than 'doing' complementary therapy-based interventions. Being comfortable with less 'doing' but rather 'being with' may present therapists with challenges. Having had a 'no' response to an offer of massage or other intervention may feel like a rejection of help, but is also an assertion that this may not be appreciated at a given time (see Case study 6.3). Some patients may also be reluctant to receive treatments due to fatigue, current discomfort and a lack of exposure to touch therapies or even a less than helpful prior experience. All patients must be asked to give their consent to interventions on the proviso that they can stop and adjust the treatment and/or position at any point.

Case study 6.3: A shift from 'doing' to 'being with'

Previously, William received 'enjoyable' massages from the team, but, on this occasion, he declined because of pain; his palliative radiotherapy was completed on the previous day. When the therapist enquired about his pain management, he explained that the medication changes had just been made and he was hoping the pain would ease. He also shared his anxieties about his limited mobility and ability to go home. On discussion, he said that the physiotherapists had been earlier and he had only managed to walk a few steps. The therapist asked, 'Do you think that once the pain has eased you will be able to walk a little further tomorrow?' He nodded and the therapist reassured him that he would only be discharged when both pain and mobility were manageable for him (this had been stated at the multidisciplinary team meeting earlier in the day).

The therapist adjusted his pillows and ensured there was water on the table within his reach. William expressed his appreciation of the time taken to talk through his concerns. The therapist documented and reported William's concern about discharge to his palliative care specialist nurse. The next day William requested a massage, 'Because of all the walking I've done today.' He was happily discharged three days later.

Importantly, recruiting experienced and skilled therapists to an SPC role is essential; there needs to be a level of professional autonomy and ability to interact with the wider multidisciplinary team. In addition, all therapists must have access to clinical supervision (see Chapter 3).

As a space for receiving evidence-based medical care, delivered by highly trained and role-defined professionals in clean, well-lit rooms, a clinical environment can at its best be safe and, at its worst, dehumanizing. The provision of therapies, such as massage, delivered by non-clinical staff or supervized volunteers provides patients and carers with contact that is concerned with comfort, rather than treatment. Inevitably, when funds are required, policies are being developed, or interventions reviewed for acceptability by the wider team, evidence of effectiveness may be demanded. Randomized controlled double-blinded trials do not fit the paradigm of the interactive, adapted and tactile nature of most touch-based therapies (see Chapter 5). A service evaluation or review is a valuable exercise, not only for the team but also to contribute towards knowledge about developing services in complex areas of care.

The focus of the three-year review was patients, although the team also provided carers with complementary therapies. A future audit/review would require palliative care-specific data to be collected with carers. For example, the team utilized a simple ten-point visual analogue scale – the Wellbeing Thermometer, devised by Field (2000) in studies with carers (see Chapter 14). Family members, carers and friends, with some informal training and support from trained therapists, have the potential in their hands (and hearts) to change the ambience and extend the 'circle of care' providing simple interventions (Goldschmidt and van Meines 2012).

One published evaluation or review of an acute cancer service, which provides a range of interventions to help with medical procedures/treatment, went beyond the treatment record sheets in terms of data collection (Mackereth *et al.* 2015). A researcher, not involved in patient care, interviewed both patients and carers so as to reduce the bias associated with giving feedback post-treatment. This review proposal was submitted for ethical approval. The concern was that when interviewees were being asked in-depth questions, emotional feelings might be revealed to someone who was not directly involved in their care. The interviews did trigger emotional release for two carers, whose partners were at the end of life, but both reported feeling calmer from sharing their experiences.

Therapists at a cancer care centre have contributed to qualitative studies about supervision, providing therapies to the opposite sex in a clinical setting and training (McLaren *et al.* 2014; Mackereth *et al.* 2010). It would be helpful to more fully explore the experience of being a palliative care specialist therapist. The demographic detail from the retrospective review of treatment records was limited. An economic review was not included as the service was charity funded and the purpose was to improve/assist with quality of life and wellbeing.

SUMMARY

A wealth of knowledge and skills in working with palliative care and in end-of-life situations has evolved from this project. It would be useful to widen the evaluation to other acute palliative care settings to gather information about evolving complementary therapy provision. Suggestions for service evaluations and reviews are as follows:

- Develop patient and carer documentation, which enables you to record essential information for legal, reflective and therapeutic reasons and to inform service evaluations and reviews (see Chapter 4).

- Recognize that feedback to the therapist, although anecdotal, may provide valuable anonymized quotes for presentations and reports.

- Consider including a simple measure to rate an issue or concern pre- and post-treatment, or through a series of treatments, to assess both the value of the work and to provide data for service evaluations.

- Store/utilize/dispose of any confidential documentation/ electronic patient/carer information in accordance with clinical governance and legal requirements.

- When sharing your work, its successes and challenges, ensure patient/carer confidentiality at all times, for example no biographical details, and use only composite case studies.

- Prepare short versions of service evaluation reports for distribution to participants involved in service evaluations and patient groups.

- Consider preparing service evaluation reports for publication, eliciting the support and agreement from your manager and/ or academic and audit departments.

REFERENCES

Andrews, G. and Mackereth, P. (2012) 'Age, sex, disease, ethnicity et al. – are complementary therapies reaching the parts? ' *Complementary Therapies in Cancer Care 18:* 2–3.

Beck, I., Runeson, I., Blomqvist, K. (2009) 'To find inner peace: soft massage as an established and integrated part of palliative care.' *International Journal of Palliative Nursing 15,* 11, 541–545.

Cronfalk, B.S., Ternestedt, B-M., Strang, P. (2009) 'Soft tissue massage: early intervention for relatives whose family members died in palliative cancer care.' *Journal of Clinical Nursing 19,* 7–8, 1040–1048.

Department of Health (2005) *Research Governance for Health and Social Care.* London. DoH.

Field, T. (2000) *Touch Therapy.* London. Churchill Livingstone.

Gerrish, K. and Mawson, S. (2005) 'Research, audit, practice development and service evaluation: implications for research and clinical governance.' *Practice Development in Health Care; 4,* 1, 33–39.

Goldschmidt, B. and van Meines, N. (2012) Comforting Touch in Dementia and End of Life Care: Take My Hand. Philadelphia PA: Singing Dragon.

Mackereth, P., Hackman, E., Knowles, R., Mehrez, A. (2015) 'The value of stress relieving techniques.' *Cancer Nursing Practice 14,* 4, 14–21.

Mackereth, P., Hackman, E., Knowles, R., Mehrez, A. (2014) 'The value of complementary therapies for carers witnessing patients medical procedures.' *Cancer Nursing Practice 13,* 9, 32–38.

Mackereth, P., Bardy, J., Finnegan-John, J., Molassiotis, A. (2014) 'Receiving or not receiving acupuncture in a trial: the experience of participants recovering from breast cancer treatment.' *Complementary Therapies in Clinical Practice 20,* 4, 291–296.

Mackereth, P.A., Parkin, S., Donald, G., Antcliffe, N. (2010) 'Clinical supervision and complementary therapists: an exploration of the rewards and challenges of cancer care.' *Complementary Therapies in Clinical Practice 16,* 3, 143–148.

McLaren, N., Mackereth, P., Hackman, E., Holland, F. (2014) 'Working out of the 'toolbox': an exploratory study with complementary therapists in acute cancer care.' *Complementary Therapies in Clinical Practice 20,* 4, 207–221.

Molassiotis, A., Bardy J., Finnegan-John J., Mackereth, P. *et al.* (2012) 'Acupuncture for cancer-related fatigue in patients with breast cancer: a pragmatic randomized controlled trial.' *Journal of Clinical Oncology Dec 20,* 30, 36, 4470–4476.

Nyatanga, B. (2015) 'Using complementary therapies in palliative care.' *British Journal of Community Nursing 20,* 4, 203.

Vandergrift, A. (2013) Use of complementary therapies in hospice and palliative care. *OMEGA 67* (1–2) 227–232.

Part 2

PRACTICAL APPLICATIONS OF AROMATHERAPY, MASSAGE AND RELAXATION

Chapter 7

AROMATHERAPY
The SYMPTOM Model

Dr Peter A. Mackereth and Paula Maycock

KEY WORDS
constipation, aromatherapy, symptom, abdominal massage, peristalsis

INTRODUCTION

As aromatherapy and other complementary therapies have become popular, therapists are increasingly being asked to help with 'difficult to treat' symptoms. These requests can come from a patient's medical team, who may have thoroughly investigated the symptom and provided interventions, yet the symptom persists. It may be that contributing behavioural or psychological issues are exacerbating the symptom, which could be helped by skillful use of a complementary therapy intervention. A complementary therapist is not trained to make a medical diagnosis, but may work collaboratively with a medical team to assist in managing symptoms and disorders.

We have developed a model to structure an approach to exploring how best to assess, support and/or to refer on patients with complex symptoms, such as constipation or nausea (see Table 7.1). We have found this model to be useful in our work with a variety of patient and carer concerns. It needs to be acknowledged that a symptom rarely occurs as a singular problem; more often it is part of a cluster of physical, psychological and behavioural concerns. Cognizant of this complexity, it is important that therapists be holistic in the information gathering and assessment of a patient's wellbeing. As the therapeutic relationship develops, and trust is gained, patients often disclose to therapists more about what troubles them. Sometimes this information, and associated fears, may not have been shared with the patient's medical team. As therapists, we need to be vigilant to disclosures, their relevance to medical care and how we can best manage patient confidentiality. In this chapter, we use 'constipation' to describe the SYMPTOM model in action.

The elements of the model are outlined in Table 7.1.

Table 7.1: SYMPTOM – a model for reviewing the role of aromatherapy in symptom management

S	Symptom definition and causation. Is there a medical term to describe the symptom? Is it part of a cluster? Is it a 'red flag' for a health concern/medical emergency? Is there a psychological component to the definition? Is there a known causation?
Y	Your patient's experience of the symptom. How does he/she describe it? Is there a means of measuring the symptom, for example Visual Analogue Scale (VAS)? Is it generalized, specific to an area or activity or time of day? Are there any triggers and does it migrate to other parts of the body?
M	Medical management. Has the patient reported the symptom to medical staff? Has the symptom been investigated? Does the patient receive any medication or intervention to help with the symptom now or in the recent past? (He/she may have stopped taking the medication or be using it only occasionally.) Have you been asked/been given permission to provide aromatherapy to the patient, or is he/she self-referring? Will you or the patient report back to the medical staff?
P	Purpose of you providing aromatherapy. What are your expectations? What is the evidence of benefit? What does your patient expect from receiving aromatherapy?
T	Technique/treatment delivery/route. Assess and review method, for example aromastick, base, gel, lotion, and/or combined with acupressure, reflexology or hypnotherapy.
O	Options/advice. Ensure that this is within your professional role/organization's policy. Record and provide confidential written/electronic detail, if appropriate. You will be accountable for all aspects of the intervention(s).
M	Monitor/maintain symptom control. Ensure that the patient has a means of reporting any change or outcome of the intervention(s). If in doubt, always refer patients back to a medical practitioner. Remember, a symptom can be a warning sign of a change in their medical condition or health.

(Mackereth and Maycock 2014)

APPLYING THE SYMPTOM MODEL TO THE SYMPTOM OF CONSTIPATION

Definition of symptom and causation

Constipation is perhaps most conveniently thought of as a *symptom*. In contrast, functional constipation and secondary constipation are *disorders.* Changes in bowel habits may require investigation if they persist. When clinicians investigate health concerns they are trained to be alert to 'red flags'; these are paramount to making an assessment and triggering further investigations. Red flag symptoms may prompt a health professional to make a rapid referral to a medical specialist or, in certain circumstances, instigate attendance at an emergency care department (Candelli *et al.* 2001; Collins and O'Brien 2015). These can include:

- alternating constipation and diarrhea

- persisting nausea and vomiting

- bleeding – fresh blood and/or tarry stools

- severe abdominal pain/guarding.

Leakage of loose stool can occur around impacted faeces, with small quantities of stool being passed frequently and without sensation; this is also known as *bypass soiling*. Encopresis is an alternative term for faecal incontinence, but is rarely used in patient communication. Secondary constipation is also known as *organic constipation.* There was no agreement on diagnostic criteria and terminology until the Rome II Diagnostic Criteria for Functional Gastrointestinal Disorders (Drossman *et al.* 1999). According to the updated Rome III criteria (Shih and Kwan 2007) a patient must have experienced at least two of the following symptoms over the preceding three months:

- straining

- lumpy/hard stools

- sensation of incomplete evacuation

- sensation of anorectal blockage

- manual manoeuvering required to defecate

- fewer than three bowel movements per week.

It is important to remember that drugs which are commonly prescribed for people living with cancer can induce constipation; these can include opioids, iron, antacids, calcium and anticholinergic agents. Disease can induce constipation from, for example, direct pressure/ obstruction from a localized tumour or from spinal cord compression secondary to advanced disease. Indirectly, cachexia, immobility and low mood or depression can also compromise bowel function and appetite/ability to eat (Laugsand *et al.* 2011).

Your patient's experience

Eliciting a history of, and changes to, bowel habits is essential. Nearly 80 per cent of the population believes they should open their bowels daily, with 90 per cent believing that bowel regularity is essential for good health. Episodes of temporary constipation can occur when people are away from home, anxious or travelling. There are complications of persisting constipation made worse by straining; these can include discomfort and pain, rectal bleeding, haemorrhoids and anal fissures (Collins and O'Brien 2015). In a cancer care setting there can be complex reasons for constipation.

Medical management

It is important to know if the patient has reported the constipation to his/her doctor, so the current underlying cause can be investigated. It is therefore vital that the aromatherapist knows of these possibilities and treats within safe guidelines, and always within their own sphere of knowledge and the rules of the employing body. If you are working within a medical setting you will be adding your findings to the patient's medical notes as well as taking responsibility for your results. Dietary change and exercise are first line recommendations rather than reaching for laxatives, enemas and suppositories (Bush 2000). In particular, the latter may not address the underlying problem, but can lead to side-effects and dependency. A therapist can encourage patients to adhere to medical and dietary advice, but if conservative measures fail and the patient is clearly compliant with the advice, a more detailed evaluation should be performed by medical staff.

Purpose

Defining the purpose of your aromatherapy intervention is paramount. You may need to assist patients to uncover the underlying cause or triggers of the constipation and then work with their expectations. These should always be based on what might be achievable within your role and skill set. We have always found a reliable first port of call in managing constipation is to manage the anxiety that surrounds it. When anxiety is reduced, other concerns linked to constipation, such as fear or low mood, may be eased. It is important to set goals, which could include changing behaviours around bowel care rather than promise/claim 'regular' bowel motions (see Options/Advice later in this chapter). We have coined the term 'aromaease' to describe using aromatherapy combined with other complementary modalities to promote symptom relief. In terms of constipation this would be to promote peristalsis, reduce anxiety and low mood, improve comfort and ease effort linked to bowel movement. Integral to the 'aromaease' work is increasing the patient's awareness and understanding of influences on bowel function and processes, for example to promote peristalsis as mentioned above (see Box 7.1 and Case Study 7.1). Importantly, carers can play an important part, with the patient's ongoing consent, in delivering simple techniques and encouraging a loved one to practise a taught self-help activity (see Box 7.1 and Case study 7.2).

Techniques

It is important to remember that a therapist can provide intervention over clothed areas or parts of the body distant to the area(s) of discomfort/concern. If it is possible, and with the patient's consent, the therapist can deliver abdominal/lower back massage using base oil with or without essential oils. Therapists with additional training can advance this work by:

- considering the use of integrating acupressure points/ meridian/reflexology work

- combining hypnotherapy/guided imagery using a selected aromastick (see Chapter 8)

- using 'in the right place/at the right time' practice – associating the intervention(s) with the activity, for example toileting

- offering to teach a family member or partner the 'I Love You' abdominal massage routine, or, if a reflexologist, show how to gently work the specific bowel areas of the hands/feet.

Box 7.1: The 'I Love You' abdominal massage routine for self-massage by the patient

This routine utilizes gentle stroking. Only work in a clockwise direction.

1. Wash and dry hands.

2. Apply oil supplied by therapist.

3. Place cupped hands over tummy.

4. Scoop down left side of tummy using the heel of your hand six times - the 'I'.

5. Scoop up starting on the lower right side, then move across your tummy finishing down the left side six times (following the large bowel) – the 'L'.

6. Partially circle the umbilicus in a 'U' shape clockwise, again six times. Finish by gentle holding the tummy with cupped hands.

7. Adaptions – work the same areas over the lower back using oil; include gentle massage of upper buttocks.

8. Work either the tummy or lower back over clothes or a towel without oil. If trained as a reflexologist, utilize the hand or foot bowel/helper areas.

Note: This routine can be done by the patient while toileting (association with bowel routines). Avoid after a meal or if any areas are tender.

Self-hypnosis has been used to help patients gain control of bowel function, with evidence from the literature that emotions and mood can have a direct effect on gut motility (Taylor 2010). Listening to peristalsis is possible using an extended stethoscope or even using a natal heart monitor. Bowel movement can often be heard and even felt; the sounds of these gurgles are indicative of peristalsis. When patients are receiving welcomed comfort and touch, these sounds can become noticeably louder. Within the field of biodynamic massage therapy, these sounds are encouraged and regulated, using either massage movements or holding techniques that promote the flow of peristalsis.

There can be release of emotions and a sense of connectedness that arise after this welcomed and sensitive work (Carroll 2002).

It is worth exploring the aromatherapy and constipation literature to uncover current evidence for interventions and essential oil choices. However, our review only identified two papers, which are summarized in Box 7.2.

Box 7.2: Summaries of two studies relating to constipation

Study 1: Effect of aromatherapy massage for the relief of constipation in the elderly (Kim *et al.* 2005)

Purpose and methodology
The purpose of this study was to verify the effect of aromatherapy massage on constipation in the elderly. This study was of ten days' duration. It employed a randomized control group pre-test and post-test design. The experimental group received abdominal massage using essential oils (EOs) with rosemary, lemon and peppermint, and the control group received a placebo massage. To evaluate the effect of aromatherapy, the degree of constipation was measured using the constipation assessment scale (CAS) and the number of bowel movements per week. Data was analyzed by repeated measures of Analysis of Variance (ANOVA) using the Statistical Package for Social Sciences (SPSS) program.

Result
The score on the CAS of the experimental group was significantly lower than that of the control group. In addition, the average number of bowel movements in the experimental group was higher than that of the control group. The effect of the aromatherapy lasted two weeks after treatment, while the placebo effect lasted seven to ten days after treatment.

Conclusion
The finding of this study showed that aromatherapy helps relieve constipation in the elderly.

Study 2: Effectiveness of aroma massage on advanced cancer patients with constipation: a pilot study (Lai *et al.* 2011)

Purpose and methodology
The purpose of this study was to verify the effect of aromatherapy massage on constipation in advanced cancer patients. The method employed a randomized control group pre- and post-test design and included an aroma massage group, a plain massage group and control group. To evaluate the effect of aromatherapy, the degree of constipation was measured using the CAS, severity level of constipation and the frequency of bowel movements. Data was analyzed by repeated measures of the Mann-Whitney U test, Wilcoxon signed ranks test, Spearman's rho and ANOVA using the SPSS program.

Results
The score of the constipation assessment scale of the aroma massage group was significantly lower than that of the control group. Apart from the improvement in bowel movements, the results showed significantly improved quality of life in physical and support domains of the aroma massage group.

Conclusion
The findings of this study suggest that aroma massage can help to relieve constipation in patients with advanced cancer.

Selection was made from the following essential oils: bitter orange, black pepper, rosemary and patchouli; the base used was olive oil.

The method of administration for the treatment (massage, gel, lotion, etc.) and the blend to be used must be agreed, appropriate and convenient for patients to use. For example, we have found that a blend of essential oils in an aromastick is a popular and empowering method for introducing blends to help with insomnia, nausea and anxiety (Stringer and Donald 2011). Aromasticks could be combined with hypnotherapy, reflexology and even acupressure to help some forms of constipation (see Chapter 8 on aromasticks).

Options/Advice

Techniques are offered to patients to assist with constipation; these include abdominal massage, hand and foot massage using an appropriate and patient-preferred blend. If a therapist holds reflexology training, and has the patient's consent, he/she could work reflexology areas on the hands. Patients may have been given medical/lifestyle/ behavioural advice, but not had support in carrying out the activity or change in behaviour. An aromatherapist could review these options and advice and support patients to make the appropriate changes. If the patient is unsure about the advice then he/she can be encouraged to obtain clarification from the appropriate health professional.

Monitoring

It is useful to assess both the quality and quantity of bowel activity. A Visual Analogue Scale (VAS) scored in 0–10 centimetre sections, which features opposing terms either end of the continuum, could be used. For example, the opposing terms could be, 'I comfortably attempt to/open my bowels' to 'It was uncomfortable to attempt to/ open my bowels.' It is useful to ask, 'How frequently do you open your bowels in a week?' Be careful about being tied to bowel movement outcomes. It maybe more appropriate in the palliative and supportive care setting to consider comfort, anxiety linked to bowel movements or even achieving a satisfactory release of wind/flatus.

THE SYMPTOM MODEL IN PRACTICE

To illustrate how the model has been applied in practice, descriptors of two case histories can be found below, together with a reflective statement.

Case study 7.1: A single 'getting going' session

Symptom/medical management: David was recovering from bowel surgery, which included formation of a temporary colostomy. David had had no bowel movement since surgery, three days previously.

Your patient's experience: David reported tension in his neck and a headache, and he felt very conscious of everything going on around him.

Purpose: David was offered interventions (including self-help techniques) to promote relaxation and parasympathetic action (for example peristalsis).

Techniques/Options: To support self-help, the therapist demonstrated a simple hand massage combined with an aromastick. David selected one that reminded him of his garden. He was encouraged to self-massage and use the aromastick three times a day.

Monitoring: During the session, David reported 'rumblings' audible to the therapist and an awareness of thirst. This was an opportunity to encourage David to drink to hydrate the stools and help with their passage. He requested that the therapist return in two days. However, feedback from the nurses included that his stoma had worked, and therefore he had been discharged.

Reflection

During a gentle foot massage, David talked about his former work as a manager, the shock of diagnosis and his unfamiliarity (and lack of privacy) within hospital. The therapist talked about promoting peristalsis through relaxation, listening for tummy gurgles and the importance of bowel movement to his recovery. David was very interested in the mechanics of the gut and links to the nervous system.

Case study 7.2: A comfy tummy with massage and guided imagery

Symptom/medical management: Sandra had breast cancer and lung and bone metastasis. She was receiving oxygen therapy and pain relief via a syringe driver plus patches. Sandra was also provided with laxatives.

Your patient's experience: Sandra talked about being breathless on exertion, confined to bed with poor appetite and being uncomfortable when sitting on the commode for any length of time.

Purpose: To promote comfort and relaxation during the use of the commode.

Techniques/Options: Sandra was offered massage movements in the form of a simple 'I Love You' on her tummy and lower back. With Sandra's agreement, this approach was also demonstrated to her daughter. A grape seed oil base, plus sweet orange essential oil (chosen by the patient) was used. During the massage, the therapist provided a short visualization using the metaphor of a 'comfy' train or other vehicle travelling to a preferred destination using the senses, for example variable countryside, different season/temperature, time of day, sounds, movement, aromas, etc. (see Chapter 11, Guided Imagery).

Monitoring: Sandra reported that her comfort was improved by having her therapist (or her daughter) massage her lower back, while she was sitting on the commode.

Reflection

Aside from the feedback from Sandra, her daughter requested massage to help her at this time, disclosing during the session that she wanted to make the most of her time with her mum. Providing the massages for her mum made her feel 'especially' close and important to her care. Sandra drifted into unconsciousness and died during the night the following week.

SUMMARY

The SYMPTOM model can be used as a means of exploring concerns raised by a patient, with the intention of aiding an aromatherapist to review his/her knowledge of a specific symptom and the purpose of aromatherapy. Using a structured approach can also assist teachers of aromatherapy in preparing presentations and group work activity for students.

REFERENCES

Bush, S. (2000) 'Fluids, Fiber and Constipation.' *Nursing Times Plus 96*, 31, 11–12.

Candelli, M., Nista, E. C., Zocco, M.A., Gasbarrini, A. (2001) 'Idiopathic chronic constipation: pathophysiology, diagnosis and treatment.' *Hepato-gastroenterology 48*, 40, 1050–1057.

Carroll, R. (2002) 'Biodynamic Massage in Psychotherapy: Reintegrating, Re-owning and Re-associating Through the Body.' In T. Staunton (ed.) *Body Psychotherapy*. Hove, East Sussex: Brunner-Routledge.

Collins, B.R. and O'Brien, L. (2015) 'Prevention and management of constipation in adults.' *Nursing Standard 29*, 32, 49–58.

Drossman, D., Corazziari, E., Talley, N. J., Thompson, W. G. *et al.* (1999) *Rome II: A Multinational Consensus Document on Functional Gastrointestinal Disorders.* Gut 45 Supplement II.

Kim, M.A.I., Sakong, J.K., Kim, E.J., Kim, E.H. (2005) 'Effect of aromatherapy massage for the relief of constipation in the elderly.' *Taehan Kanho Hakhoe Chi 35*, 1, 56–64. (Translation).

Lai, T.K.I., Cheung, M.C., Lo. C.K., Ng, K.L. *et al.* (2011) 'Effectiveness of aroma massage on advanced cancer patients with constipation: a pilot study.' *Complementary Therapies in Clinical Practice 17,* 1, 37–43.

Laugsand, E., Jakobsen, G., Kaasa, S., Klepstadp, P. (2011) 'Inadequate symptom control in advanced cancer patients across Europe.' *Supportive Care in Cancer 19,* 12, 2005–2014.

Mackereth, P. and Maycock, P. (2014) 'Aromatherapy and the SYMPTOM model. *In Essence 13* 3, 9–12.

Shih, D. and Kwan, L. (2007) 'All roads lead to Rome: Update on Rome 111 Criteria and new treatment options.' *The Gastroenterology Report 1,* 2, 56–65.

Stringer, J. and Donald, G. (2011) 'Aromasticks in cancer care: an innovation not to be sniffed at.' *Complementary Therapies in Clinical practice 116,* 21, 9–15.

Taylor, E. (2010) 'Hypno-psychotherapy for Functional Gastro-intestinal Disorders.' In A. Cawthorn and P. Mackereth (eds) *Integrative Hypnotherapy: Complementary Approaches in Clinical Care.* London: Churchill Livingstone.

Chapter 8

AROMASTICKS
A Portable Aromatic Powerhouse
Paula Maycock, Dr Peter A. Mackereth and Ann Carter

KEY WORDS
aromasticks, mother blend, inhalation, anchoring, sensory language

INTRODUCTION

We have found aromasticks to be helpful in many areas of clinical practice, and in this chapter we would like to share with you some of the lessons we have learned in making the most of their use. On our training courses, over recent years, we have met many aromatherapists, who, having been introduced to aromasticks, would like to use them in both clinical and private practice. As there is little in the way of instruction on how to optimize their use, aromatherapists have been left to their own devices to figure out how to get the most out of using an aromastick.

This chapter will cover the principles and practice of using aromasticks in clinical settings. These include the rationale for blending and creating 'mother blends', as well as hygiene and safety. Key therapeutic issues are explored; these include the processes of dispensing and 'installing' the aromasticks, increasing potency through 'anchoring', as well as instructions for aftercare.

INHALATION OF ESSENTIAL OILS AS A THERAPEUTIC APPROACH

The nasal route and respiratory interface can be the most effective means for the delivery and absorption of essential oils (Battaglia 2004, first published 1995). Inhalation may give a speed of absorption, which rivals intravenous administration, even with the presence of the physical barrier of mucus. As this is a very fast method of uptake, inhalation is particularly useful when seeking to engage, soothe and calm a distressed individual. The patient's perception of the blend's aroma is important in engaging with and supporting patient compliance. The significance of prior life experience and the link to smell memory is also important. For example, the memory scent of alcohol-based skin wipes, used during cannulation, may evoke nausea or vomiting. This response is in complete contrast to recalling the aromas of flowers at a wedding, which may trigger a recollection of joy and celebration.

Initially, our experience of using the inhalation route began by putting essential oil combinations on a tissue for immediate use by a patient during stressful procedures. However, the possibilities of using essential oils through inhalation were transformed with the advent of aromasticks. The advantages of using an aromastick are:

- the shape and size of the aromastick make it easy and safe to handle

- the aroma does not disperse throughout a space, such as a ward or a four-bedded bay

- a choice can easily be made from a selection of prepared blends already contained inside the aromastick

- it is a takeaway product for the sole use of the person for whom it is prescribed.

THE STRUCTURE OF AN AROMASTICK

Rather than putting essential oils onto a tissue or cottonwool ball, the essential oils are offered to the patient on a wick, which is enclosed within a plastic tube. This tube is perforated at one end to allow the aroma to be detected when sniffed. The prepared stick has an outer cover that limits the evaporation of the oils and makes the stick portable (see Figure 8.1). When prepared by an aromatherapist, the essential oil blend can be customized to include oils with claimed benefits for the alleviation of anxiety, nausea and insomnia. Some cancer care centres have also developed and evaluated the use of aromasticks, focused on alleviating specific symptoms (Dyer 2008, 2013).

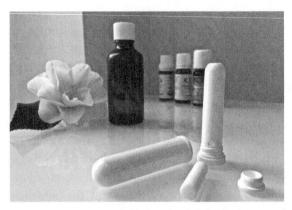

*Figure 8.1: An aromastick showing the wick (in the foreground)
and the container; the seal is on the right-hand side*

It is possible to create and modify blends to include particular patient preferences for an aroma, thus helping to maximize compliance with this treatment. We routinely use aromasticks to help patients with stressful procedures, such as scans, cannulation and radiotherapy (especially where the wearing of a restrictive mask is likely for patients with head and neck cancers), and to assist in smoking cessation work (Mackereth and Maycock 2010). When given to patients in such acutely stressful situations, aromasticks can assist in achieving and sustaining a calm state. The use of an aromastick can be incorporated within another intervention for a synergistic effect, such as guided imagery or The HEARTS Process (see Chapters 11 and 12). With training and supervision guided by an appropriate standard operating procedure (see Chapter 4), therapists without prior aromatherapy qualifications can offer aromasticks as part of their therapeutic toolbox.

MAKING THE 'MOTHER BLEND'

Aromatherapists will make blends for patients in several different ways, depending on their training and personal preferences. The blends can be as flexible and as creative as you wish, depending on your work situation and the purpose for creating the blends. Initially, our blends were developed from the practical experience of aromatherapists in the complementary therapy team. Following feedback and outcomes from patients and clinical staff, we formulated a few blends that were found to be most valued by the patients. Safety aspects and how patients might use them were considered, so the aromasticks could be introduced to the service in a managed and audited way.

To maximize patient choice, we developed six blends: two were designed to help with anxiety, two to help with sleep and two to help with nausea. Patients have reported that symptoms are made worse by their anxiety (Stringer and Donald 2011), so we focused on blends that were popular and which helped to reduce anxiety and promoted relaxation and feelings of comfort. Currently, the two blends designed to help with anxiety are offered as the first option; if neither of the 'anxiety blends' are liked, or are found to be unsuitable for an individual, a third blend is offered. Rejecting blends is a key process for engaging the patient in taking charge of the intervention. In some ways, this is like 'trying it on for size'; the preferred option is given additional status, and a sense of ownership is enhanced by the rejection of the other two.

The essential oils used in blends must also be acceptable for use in your workplace; create blends that are popular, affordable and made up in quantities that will be used, rather than 'sitting on the shelf'. A typical blend contains three or four essential oils suitable for the emotional and physical symptoms being addressed. To avoid the association of a specific aroma with a stressful process/event, such as cannulation, the individual components of the blend should not be identifiable. In our experience, patients will frequently suggest the identity of the different oils in a blend and ask, 'Is there some lavender in there?' This is understandable and we usually explain that the oils in a blend have been formulated to complement each other and the aroma may change over time. We don't agree or disagree with what the patient perceives – we simply ask if the patient enjoys the aroma that is reminiscent of lavender.

EXAMPLES OF ESSENTIAL OILS WE USE IN BLENDS FOR PATIENTS

Typically, we include three or four essential oils from the following: citrus bergamia (bergamot), boswellia carterii (frankincense), citrus limon (lemon), citrus reticulata (mandarin), lavandula angustifolia (lavender), styrax benzoin (benzoin), piper nigrum (black pepper) and elettaria cardamomum (cardamom). In spite of the expense, we may include citrus aurantium (neroli) or melissa officianalis (melissa) in our blends. These more expensive oils are not used in large quantities and only when an individual situation requires their use. When expensive essential oils are included in a blend, we reduce the volume of the 'mother blend' made. A favourite original blend of one of the authors was to use bergamot and frankincense in a ratio of one to one. At a later date, our refinement was the inclusion of benzoin, a component of over-the-counter treatments for chest and sinus problems. The addition of benzoin reminded some patients of the aroma of vanilla, which had comforting associations.

THE ROLE OF 'MOTHER BLENDS'

For reasons of accuracy and convenience, we normally make and store blends as 30–50 ml (milliletres) volumes of 'mother blend'. The wick of the aromastick is loaded with 1 ml from the 'mother blend'. This equates to approximately 20 drops of blend and we find this gives 'good volume' for the wick size. A 'mother blend' allows for reproducibility; this is also essential for any research work on blend efficacy for particular situations and symptoms. The essential oils are measured in millilitres rather than in drops, to provide accuracy and consistency. Using a mother blend is particularly useful as it increases the ease and speed at which the aromastick can be constructed; at the same time it increases accuracy and consistency, which is much easier than counting drops from individual bottles.

After application to the wick, the longevity of the aroma depends on both the chemistry of the blend and how the aromastick is stored. Ideally, when the blend has been applied to the wick, it should have a 'useful working life' of at least two months when stored in a cool, dark place. This allows patients to continue using the aromastick when required, away from the hospital, clinic or hospice. Highly volatile blends, such as those with high citrus oil content, usually oxidize or evaporate quickly and so may have short-term use. The addition of middle and base notes will help to increase blend longevity (Price and Price 2011, first published 1995).

SAFETY CHECKS

When choosing the essential oils for an aromastick blend there are cautions to be considered. For example, where a patient is known to have asthma, or other breathing problems, the aromastick should not be used prior to, or immediately after, the use of nebulized or 'puffer' delivered drugs. It is important for aromatherapists to be aware of the patient's drug regime to ensure that essential oils do not accentuate or reduce the action of medication. We gain consent from patients for the use of aromasticks, providing an information leaflet to support verbal instruction. We advise caution in situations with patients where consent may be unclear. For example, offering an aromastick to patients under the age of 16, or to patients living with learning difficulties may require parental/guardian involvement. Particular care should also be observed when gaining consent for their use with patients living with a form of dementia and memory loss. For hygiene and convenience purposes, the aromasticks can be individually packaged, combined with an information leaflet, in a small, clean plastic bag. In addition to the instructions on the use of the aromastick, the leaflet should include contact information, in case patients have any queries or concerns. Our instruction sheet reiterates that the aromastick is for the patient's use only – see below.

AN EASY WAY OF USING AROMASTICKS WITH PATIENTS

We have found the following framework a useful way to help patients make effective use of aromasticks. We give patients a similar sheet to take home or to refer to at a later time.

Making effective use of your aromastick

- This aromastick has been blended to support you. Please do not share it as the essential oil blend was selected for your use only.

- First, unscrew the cover from the wick holder.

- Hold the stick with the perforated end towards your nose, between two and three inches away from your nostrils. Do not insert the tube into your nose.

- Breathe in through your nose in a steady comfortable breath. (This allows the vapour to be absorbed within your nose.)

- Breathe out through your mouth so you do not blow the plant oil vapour out again.

- Repeat this comfortable in/out breathing twice more.

- This set of three comfortable breaths is an easy and comfortable way for you to benefit from using your aromastick.

- Repeat the breathing technique when required, as discussed with your therapist.

- Remember to close the aromastick tightly after use.

- Regularly clean the stick with a clean, damp cloth or tissue.

- Do not immerse the aromastick in any fluids.

- If you have any queries contact…(insert therapist contact details).

- If you have any concerns, stop using the aromastick and contact…(insert therapist contact details).

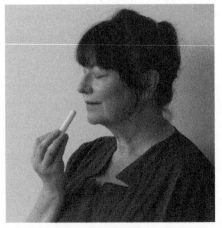

Figure 8.2: Demonstrating the use of an aromastick

UNDERSTANDING THE PROCESS OF 'ANCHORING'

An anchor is a 'stimulus' that is linked to and triggers a psychological state (O'Connor and Seymour 2002). Everyone has good and bad memories of life events that can be anchored or linked to certain stimuli. For example, a common anchor may be music that has personal meaning and evokes an emotion. The emotion can be enhanced or decreased by the degree of attention we give to the music and other factors, such as the volume or remembering the context. Being covered with a warm towel can also create a positive response, arousing memories of being nurtured as a child. Seeing a picture of a place associated with happy memories can immediately effect physiological changes in the body, producing 'feel-good' sensations.

APPLICATIONS OF 'ANCHORING' IN CLINICAL PRACTICE

Some therapists have told us that they typically give patients an aromastick to 'sniff' and leave it at that. However, we have found that the use of aromasticks is enhanced if patients are helped to learn an easy process which deliberately links the aroma to a pleasant experience; this approach enables patients to utilize the aromastick effectively as a self-soothing intervention (Maycock *et al.* 2014). An example from this practice is described in Case study 8.1.

Case study 8.1: Associating an aroma with positive experiences

Bob had been diagnosed with lung cancer and was waiting to have some tests. He was agitated and pacing up and down, when a nurse noticed that Bob was showing signs of hyperventilating. She approached him and Bob confided that he was angry with himself 'for being a wimp'. 'After all,' he said, 'I'm a man; I have tattoos and everything. I should be able to deal with this.' A therapist working in the clinic was asked to provide support. She offered a choice of three aromasticks and demonstrated to Bob how he could use the one he chose. Bob commented, 'It reminds me of the chest rub my mother used when I was ill with bronchitis as a child. It makes me feel she's here with me and helping me. I can wrap my hand around her (i.e. the aromastick) and hold on tight. It's such a relief to feel better and back in control.'

Bob linked the aroma immediately to his mother, and was able to articulate the comforting connection. In situations where patients are unable to make a link, or to sustain it, the aromastick risks being put away without further thought. Our experience of purposefully 'anchoring' the aroma of the blend to something pleasant assists in the calming process and offers a means of enhancing and sustaining the connection. We suggest that by reinforcing the link, the effects of the aromastick can become more and more potent. Steps to achieve this can include engaging with the aromastick while experiencing a pleasant or comfortable activity; for example, being with loved ones, friends, family and pets.

USING SENSORY LANGUAGE TO ANCHOR THE EFFECTIVE USE OF AROMASTICKS

The principles of using sensory language in guided imagery are explained in Chapter 11. We have found the use of sensory language to be both effective and supportive when integrated with the use of aromasticks.

When using sensory language to assist the patient to anchor an aromastick to a pleasant experience, we start by asking the person to think of an experience that he/she would be comfortable to access. Using a framework of sensory language, we can then explore this positive experience in terms of what he/she can see, hear and feel (see Chapter 11, Guided Imagery). At the end of each 'sensory stage', we ask the individual to, 'Breathe in through your nose and breathe out through your mouth,' while the patient accesses the pleasant sensory experience associated with the image.

Case study 8.2 illustrates how to combine sensory language and the use of an aromastick to first maximize the positive experience of a pleasant aroma, and second promote a deepening of the calming effects each and every time the aromastick is used. This approach enables patients to build resources in self-soothing promoted by the aromastick (Maycock *et al.* 2014).

USING IMAGERY WITH AROMASTICKS TO HELP CHANGE EMOTIONAL STATES

Some of the emotional states experienced by patients include fear, anxiety, tension, and worry. These states are experienced internally by the patient, although they cannot be physically touched by an outsider. However, they still have a sensory structure and the experience is usually stored using that structure. If we use fear as an example, the fear is likely to have colour, or a shape, or it may make a sound and have a sensation. It is also likely it will have a place somewhere in the body. The patient is unlikely to have any knowledge of the details; however, it is likely that that he/she will subconsciously be storing the emotion in this detail. Changing an emotional state in this context relies on the principle that if you change the initial structure the experience of the emotion will also change. An example is given in Case study 8.2.

Case study 8.2: Janice's magic wand

Janice was attending her third session of chemotherapy. She was anxious and fearful about the insertion of a needle to deliver her treatment. Although she could recognize how she felt she had no resources to deal with the fear. Using sensory language and asking one question at a time the therapist asked:

'What colour is the fear?'

'Does the fear have any sound?'

'Where do you feel it in your body?'

Janice told the therapist, 'It's vivid red.'

'It has a gnawing sound.'

'It's coming from here in my guts.'

The therapist then asked a second series of questions, still linked to the senses but focusing on changing the experience.

'What colour would be the opposite of the red?'

'What would be a contrast to the gnawing?'

'Where would you send the feeling away from your guts?'

Immediately, Janice said, 'It would be golden yellow.'

'It would have a gentle stroking feeling.'

'It would go out through my big toes.'

First, Janice was invited to think of drawing in the colour 'golden yellow' and to send it to 'gently stroke her tummy'. The therapist invited her to see the colour 'vivid red' 'flowing out through her "fabulous toes" and being replaced by the "golden yellow"'. At each stage of accessing the 'more positive experience' Janice accessed the 'new and more resourceful state' as she took a breath in from her aromastick. The intravenous needle was inserted in one easy movement, which Janice appeared to not notice.

COMMENTARY: JANICE'S MAGIC WAND

Janice's magic wand demonstrates another approach to helping a patient access a more positive state using her own resources; this method can be used in an acute situation with a patient undergoing a medical procedure. The therapist's aim was to help the patient find the 'more resourceful state' by changing the structure of the emotion 'fear'.

When using this approach the information that a patient gives you will sometimes sound completely illogical. Do not be tempted to suggest alternatives that make sense to you. The language used must be that of the patient, not the therapist. If you suggest a word such as 'comfy' or 'tummy' to suggest a potential state change, always check out the patient's verbal and non-verbal reactions. Some patients may not like a particular word and would prefer you to use one which he/she has suggested. When you ask a question about sensory experience, be confident that it will sound as though this is a perfectly ordinary thing to do. We have yet to meet someone who does not respond when asked an apparently unusual question about the sensory structure of an emotion. Encourage the patient to create his/her own solution and be engaged in the therapeutic activity – it is a joint venture of discovery. Importantly, encourage your patient to see themselves as the expert on their feelings. Asking just a few key questions (rather than a great long list) can help patients to explore feelings safely and in a structured way. Do not be surprised if patients report other positive outcomes. For example, pain alleviation may be their chosen outcome, but they may also report an improvement in mood or sleep patterns.

SUMMARY

We have found aromasticks to be invaluable in our work. They are portable, easy to use and offer an approach which will remind patients of their ability to self-calm and to lessen their discomfort when they choose. Aromasticks should always be enjoyed by patients or they will not use them...their noses know best. The suggestions for the essential oils given in this chapter are examples and are not intended to be an exhaustive list. Sensory language has proved invaluable in helping patients to anchor the good feelings experienced from using an aromastick. This 'resourceful' technique has encouraged individuals to continue using the aromastick while on a ward, at home and before procedures that they have found difficulty with in the past. As the patient's confidence in using the aromastick develops, so its potency is enhanced. As therapists, repeatedly seeing and hearing about the powerful effects of such a portable and easy-to-use aromatherapy tool adds to our confidence in offering it to more and more patients.

REFERENCES

Battaglia, S. (2004) *The Complete Guide to Aromatherapy.* 2nd edition. London: Perfect Potions.

Dyer, J. (2008) 'A snap-shot survey of current practice: the use of aromasticks for symptom management.' *International Journal of Clinical Aromatherapy 5,* 2, 17–21.

Dyer. J. (2013) 'The use of aromasticks at a cancer centre: a retrospective audit.' *Complementary Therapies in Clinical Practice 20,* 4, 203–206.

Mackereth, P. and Maycock, P. (2010) 'Anxiety and Panic States: the CALM Model.' In A. Cawthorn and P. Mackereth (eds) *Integrative Hypnotherapy: Complementary Approaches in Clinical Care.* London: Churchill Livingstone.

Maycock, P., Mackereth, P., Mehrez, A., Tomlinson, L. *et al.* (2014) 'Self-soothing in a tube.' *International Therapist 109,* 21–23.

O'Connor, J. and Seymour, J. (2002) *Introducing Neuro Linguistic Programming.* London: Element.

Price, S. and Price, L. (2011) *Aromatherapy for Health Professionals.* 4th edition. London: Elsevier.

Stringer, J. and Donald, G. (2011) 'Aromasticks in cancer care: an innovation not to be sniffed at.' *Complementary Therapies in Clinical Practice 116,* 21, 9–15.

Chapter 9

MALODOUR

The Potential Use of Essential Oils

Paula Maycock, Dr Peter A. Mackereth, Anita Mehrez and Dr Jacqui Stringer

KEY WORDS

odour, fungating wounds, essential oils, olfactory system

INTRODUCTION

Patients who are living with cancer can develop clinical issues such as fungating tumours that produce odours, which are difficult to eradicate. This chapter will explore the management of odour in wards and hospice settings. The content will critically review some of the solutions suggested, and explore the potential and limitations of using essential oils. The focus for the case studies is fungating malignant wounds (FMWs), which present challenges for patients, carers and staff. It must be noted that this chapter's purpose is to debate the issues rather than to provide a solution to fit all situations.

YOUR NOSE KNOWS BEST

The olfactory system is our most primitive sense. It is closely linked to the limbic system and, as such, impacts on mood and emotions. Repugnant smells can rapidly set up a negative association that can be overwhelming and distressing. Crucially, odours, aptly termed 'stench', act as a warning against health risks, such as infections or food contamination in the environment. We are literally 'wired' to be revolted by such smells and to avoid the source at all costs. Conversely, certain aromas, particularly those linked to nature, enjoyable food, or a perfume worn by a loved one, can create positive emotions and trigger pleasant and comforting associations, for example a mother's perfume (see Chapter 8, Aromasticks: A Portable Aromatic Powerhouse).

If a patient has lived with an odour for a long time, he or she may lose awareness of the extent of the smell, for example at the end of life, yet his or her carers struggle when spending time with them. Additionally, the odour may be so repugnant and invasive that it is intrusive to other patients and their visitors. Staff working in such environments may be dealing with a distressing odour for the whole of their shift. In a qualitative study, nurses reported finding it hard to control their emotions when dressing wounds that were repellent and malodorous (Georges, Grypdonck and Dierckx de Casterle 2002). In a study concerning carers living with someone with a FMW, the participants talked about having to hide their revulsion and feelings of nausea when dressing the wound (Probst *et al.* 2012). Openly discussing a bodily odour, from wherever it emanates, can be embarrassing and distressing for patients and carers as well as clinical staff (Fleck 2006).

Despite the impact that odour can have on the wellbeing of patients, staff and carers, there is a paucity of research evaluating interventions which may help the situation. Opening windows and ensuring good hygiene are of limited use, with staff often at a loss when the odour is persistent. The authors have developed ways of using essential oils (EOs) to assist clinical staff to manage these odours (Mehrez *et al.* 2015; Stringer *et al.* 2014), but there is minimal guidance in the literature on how to use EOs safely.

CAUSES OF MALODOUR

There are many clinical causes of malodour. Those described in the section below are some of the more common ones. FMWs occur when a tumour erupts through the skin and are a complication caused by the extension of a primary tumour, recurrence or metastatic spread. The FMW presents as a cauliflower-shaped lesion or as an ulcerative crater. Physical symptoms of FMW include pain, bleeding and profuse exudate, which can be foul smelling and will often harbour anaerobic bacteria (Stringer *et al.* 2014). Anaerobic and aerobic bacteria thrive and proliferate in areas of tissue where there is loss of vascularity and ulceration (Grocott 2007). The most common areas for FMWs are the breast, neck, chest, genitalia and head (Probst, Arber and Faithfull 2013).

There is a range of oral and gut conditions, including yeast infection, dental caries, gum diseases, ulcers, constipation and bowel obstruction, that can be associated with severe halitosis. Malodour can also arise from chest and urinary tract infections, with tissues, sputum pots and urine bags or bottles all being sources of odour. Diarrhea and urinary incontinence can lead to odours, particularly when hygiene is not attended to and patients are not promptly given a change of clothing or bedding. When reflecting on difficult symptoms, Corner (2008, first published 2005) describes the case study of Anne, who asked to be sedated and to not have visitors in her last days, due to severe diarrhea from a recto-vaginal fistula.

Malodour can have sources other than the patient. Carers may not want to leave the bedside for self-care, such as washing, because of the critical condition of their loved one. Some carers or staff may be unaware of body odour, halitosis and contamination of clothing from cigarette smoke, alcohol or garlic-rich food. Masking odours with heavy perfumes can add to smells, exacerbating the problem rather than disguising it. Being attended to by a staff member, whose body odour or breath is foul, can be distressing. Patients may feel unable to complain; they may disguise their discomfort and distress, even when the odour is exacerbating existing nausea and anxiety. Carers, colleagues or managers will often find it difficult to raise the issue of odour for fear of giving offence.

DISTRESS OF ODOUR

For patients, malodour can cause shame and embarrassment, curtailing intimacy and physical contact with partners and family (da Costa Santos, de Mattos and Nobre 2010). They may suffer depression and be reluctant to socialize, withdraw from travelling and thus become isolated (Stringer *et al.* 2014). Distress to carers and staff attending a patient with malodour is almost universal, particularly as the smell can be amplified when dressings are changed, or even when the patient moves (Probst, Arber and Faithfull 2013). Increasingly, patients are living longer with metastatic disease and FMWs. They need to be kept clean, with strategies to limit and control malodour. Persisting odour, particularly at the end of life, is distressing for the patient and family who might be reluctant to leave the bedside (see Case study 9.1).

INTERNET SUGGESTIONS TO BE AVOIDED

The following are some of the suggestions made by health professionals online; all are potentially hazardous but demonstrate the desperation of staff trying to tackle this challenging issue. They include leaving burnt toast or a stack of extinguished matches in a side room; both are unpleasant and considered an unacceptable health and safety risk. Placing a fresh tray of cat litter under the patient's bed daily has been proposed. Litter pellets are designed for odour control where there is physical contact, so would be ineffective for the absorption of an airborne aroma. The copious use of bathroom sprays day and night are suggested, yet aerosol sprays are banned in many hospitals for health and safety reasons.

USING ESSENTIAL OILS TO MANAGE ODOUR

Essential oils, depending on their volatility, concentration and the presence of a heat source, can release varying degrees of aroma into the environment. Absorption of smells occurs via the olfactory system through receptors in the upper nasal and oral mucosa. Odour molecules are transformed into chemical signals, which pass to limbic brain structures including the hypothalamus, the hippocampus and the amygdala, all of which can have an effect on mood and the emotions (Bensouilah and Buck 2006). There are numerous studies showing that odours such as orange, lavender and rose can have direct effects on neuropsychological and autonomic functioning in human and animal studies (Bradley *et al.* 2007; Lehrner *et al.* 2005). Robust evidence of mood improvement has been found with lemon oil compared with water controls (Kiecolt-Glaser *et al.* 2008).

ENVIRONMENTAL MANAGEMENT OF MALODOUR

There are challenges to using EOs in the atmosphere. Guidelines often prohibit the use of burners and fan/electrical aromatic diffusers due to concerns about fire risk in the presence of oxygen. Additionally, some patients may experience sensitivity to EOs with respiratory, skin and eye irritation. The combination of malodour and the use of EOs via a diffuser may be unpleasant for patients/staff (Tavares 2011). Putting a few drops of essential oil directly on bedding, while simple, risks possible skin contact irritation and sensitivity and the problem of 'aroma-overload' for the patient. Placing EOs in sprays, to be used over the top of dressings, clothes and bedding, carries the risk of the dispersed oils coming in contact with skin and eyes during spraying. Additionally, with wound dressings containing charcoal, any saturating moisture would lessen their effectiveness (Grocott 2007).

A simple approach is to provide EOs on cottonwool balls in a screw-top container, which can be opened periodically (see Figure 9.1). Introducing the blend as 'calming scent' can be a less obtrusive way of describing the 'aroma pot' to the patient and carers (Mehrez *et al.* 2015). Examples of EOs used this way (usually three oil blends) include the following: citrus bergamia, lavandula angustifolia, citrus limonum, boswellia carteri, citrus aurantium, styrax tonkinensis and eucalyptus radiata.

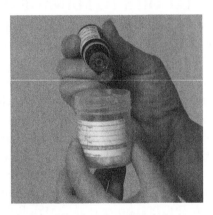

Figure 9.1: Soaking cottonwool with an essential oil blend in a small screw-top jar

A blend is advised rather than a single EO, as using one oil carries the risk of physical and emotional conditioning, associating the single aroma with the grief or trauma of current circumstances and negating its therapeutic value in the future. Acceptability of the blend should be checked a few hours after introduction and renewed with fresh oils, ideally every one or two days. Staff on later shifts should be made aware of the aroma pot in the room. The pot needs labelling, dating and a simple instruction sheet should be provided. The latter needs to include therapist contact details and instructions for disposal (for example, closing the lid and placing in the clinical waste). We advise that the instruction sheet should be laminated for ease of cleaning.

Where possible, offer patients and carers a choice of 'blended pots', unless this brings too much attention to an already difficult situation (see Chapter 8).

WOUND MANAGEMENT

Tackling the underlying cause of odour is paramount. Wound infections are a cause of malodour, which need to be managed by the medical team. Swabbing the wound may be necessary to ensure the appropriate anti-microbial treatment is provided. Metronidazole is often appropriate, and can be prescribed systemically and orally or applied topically (Paul and Pieper 2008). There are a variety of dressings available that contain activated charcoal and silver; charcoal absorbs the molecules causing malodour and silver inhibits bacterial growth (Hawthorn 2010).

However, the odour associated with FMWs is complex and standard measures are often insufficient. There are a few small, uncontrolled case series of EOs being used topically under medical supervision (see Table 9.1). Many research articles, case studies and descriptions of service provision in the literature do not report the specific variety of oils or concentration in which they were used. Some studies use commercially prepared blends or even 'scented' sprays in addition to EOs. These blends may contain ethanol and preservative, which can affect the EOs incorporated. Mercier and Knevitt (2005) reported a reduction in odour using EOs in four patients following three days of treatment, from a larger case series (n=13). Single case studies of patients with FMWs, using a combination of EOs with systemic antibiotics and chlorophyll demonstrated complete resolution of fetid odour (Warnke et al. 2004, Warnke et al. 2005). Warnke et al. (2006) have reported beneficial outcomes of EOs in the management of 30 patients living with FMWs, eradication of odour being achieved after three to four days of therapy. In a recent international survey (n=1444) the use of EOs with FMWs was reported by eight per cent of respondents; no details of specific EOs were provided (Gethin et al. 2014).

The anti-microbial effects of EOs were judged as promising by Warnke and his team (2009); they tested eucalyptus, tea tree, thyme (white), lemon, lemongrass, cinnamon, grapefruit, clove bud, sandalwood, peppermint, kunzea and sage EOs with the agar diffusion test. Exceptional inhibition zones to a range of microbes were demonstrated using four of the EOs: thyme (white), lemon, lemongrass and cinnamon, olive oil and paraffin oil, used as controls, showed no inhibition (Warnke *et al.* 2009). In cultures of pseudomonas, staphylococcus and candida albicans, silver ions used in combination with tea tree oil were found to inhibit these microbes (Low *et al.* 2011).

Marianne Tavares describes a UK hospice-based service that provided EOs (lavandula angustifolia and melaleuca alternifolia), combined with normal saline, to irrigate malodorous wounds during the period 2000–09. The 30 patients were at end of life; there were no adverse effects reported from the intervention and all had noticeable improvements in malodour (Tavares 2011).

One of the authors of this chapter has developed a cream containing EOs (novel essential oil cream or NEOC) for the management of malodour. Of additional interest was a possible additional anti-inflammatory effect and even some local tissue healing (Stringer *et al.* 2014). One of the case studies is described in Case study 9.2. Some examples of research papers relating to EOs are described in Table 9.1.

Case study 9.1: Using an 'aroma pot'

Jerry, with a history of alcohol dependency, tobacco and cannabis use, was being nursed in a side room of a ward. He had a fungating oral tumour and was at the end of life. Jerry was semi-conscious on referral and the family were keeping a vigil, concerned he might die imminently. A concern for carers, staff, other patients and their visitors was the all-pervading malodour. After receiving a call from the ward sister, a mix of three essential oils (citrus bergamia, citrus limonum and boswellia carteri), was used to create a 'calming aroma pot' by the hospital's aromatherapist; the blend was to be renewed on alternate days. Overnight, Jerry appeared more interactive, opening his eyes and squeezing the hands of his partner. The malodour was less apparent with staff opening the 'aroma pot' every one or two hours for about 10–15 minutes. Jerry died peacefully later in the night. The family were grateful for the support.

Case study 9.2: Using the novel essential oil cream

Fran presented late with breast cancer and a fungating malodorous wound and was not able to receive chemotherapy. The wound was large, malodorous and exuding excessively, requiring re-dressing a minimum of four times a day. Fran needed to be cared for in a side room and was also experiencing pain and distress. By day five of using the novel essential oil cream, the malodour was completely eradicated with much-reduced exudate, requiring dressings only to be changed on alternate days. With the odour gone, Fran's mood improved and her pain diminished and so with her agreement she moved out of the side room into a sociable four-bedded area.

Case study 9.3: Using a combined approach

Brenda was admitted to the hospice at the end of life. She had been living with a fungating breast tumour for over six months. The malodour increased with dressing changes, creating distress for Brenda and her family. The aromatherapist was asked to provide an EO cream for topical use (2.5 ml of lavandula angustifolia and melaleuca alternifolia in 100 ml cream), an 'aroma pot' (consisting of citrus bergamia, boswellia carteri and eucalyptus radiata), to be available in the room at all times and an aromastick (citrus bergamia, boswellia carteri and lavandula angustifolia) for the patient to hold or rest near her nose/mouth during dressing changes, which occurred four or five times a day. The aromastick was also used during toileting and repositioning. Brenda died during the night, four days after her admission. The malodour had reduced so the door to her room could be left open and visitors felt comfortable staying in her room.

SUMMARY

A persisting malodour in a hospital or hospice setting can be a major challenge for the patient, carers, other visitors and staff. The answers are not simple and the situation can be a delicate one, causing anxiety, distress and embarrassment to all parties. When using EOs, they must be provided with care to minimize the risks to the patient, and a choice of blend should be offered where possible. When introduced with sensitivity, aroma pots and aromasticks can be an adjunct to good nursing and medical management. Importantly, the growing use of EOs applied topically in creams and gels, or as irrigation, needs to be evaluated formally through funded research work.

Table 9.1: Details of research studies

Author	Method	Intervention	Outcome measures	Results	Comments
Warnke et al. 2004	Ongoing head and neck tumour case series using an antibacterial essential oil tumour wound rinse (n=25).	Twice a day rinse of ulcers (n=25). 5 ml mix consisted of tea tree oil, grapefruit oil, and eucalyptus oil (Megabac®) combined with standard medication of clindamycin and chlorophyll.	Clinical assessment of tumour ulcers. Feedback from patients and staff about level of malodour.	Foul smell receded within two to three days. Clinical signs of super-infection and pus were significantly reduced. Reports of pain reduction.	Uncontrolled case series with anecdotal data. No adverse reactions reported. Pain reduction attributed to anaesthetic properties of eucalyptus. Commercial preparations used in addition to EOs.
Warnke et al. 2006	Update on a case series of head and neck tumour ulcers using a new mix (n=30). See above.	Twice daily rinse of a new formula – eucalyptus-based oil mixture KMPT70, Klonemax®. Essential oils: 70 mg eucalyptus, 5 mg melaleuca, 45 mg lemongrass, 45 mg lemon, 7 mg clove leaf, 3 mg thyme on a 40% ethanol base.	Three case studies presented with photographic evidence of changes. Feedback from patients, carers and clinical staff. Bacterial swabs of ulcers.	Clinical signs of infection and malodour reduced by third and fourth day. Increased social contact with friend and relatives.	Local healing suggested possibly by the anti-inflammatory and anti-microbial effects of the commercial EO mix. No adverse effects. Further research recommended.

Study	Aim	Intervention	Measurement	Results	Conclusion
Mercier and Knevitt (2005)	Case series of a EO cream fungating wound cream (n=13).	Topical application. Patient-chosen blend with an equal amount of tea tree oil (melaleuca alternifolia) in a water-based cream at 2.5–5% dilution.	Four in-depth cases reported lavender (lavandula angustofolia) and patchouli (pogostemon cablin) added to the tea tree. Feedback from patients.	Patients reported reduced odour within days of treatment, some less exudate and bleeding. One patient said the cream was 'soothing and lovely', another 'felt better' about herself. The cream and its effects were linked to being able to go home/transfer to a care home.	Simple to use and tailored to patient preference. Further quantitative research work recommended to evaluate benefit.
Stringer et al. (2014)	To provide preliminary data for the use of a neutralizing odour cream as a management tool for symptoms of fungating malignant wounds.	A UK Foundation Trust developed NEOC, a base cream blended with essential oils to a concentration of 3%. Over an 11-month period, patients were seen for assessment of FMWs and provided with supplies of NEOC. The person responsible for dressing changes/use of NEOC carried out dressing changes as per protocol. Patients and carers were asked to evaluate the course of treatment and to grade their symptoms (n=24).	Likert scale from 0 (no problem) to 6 (worst problem ever).	The 15 patients seen more than once all reported a reduction in rating of symptoms. Three patients did not provide formal rating but annotations in their hospital notes reported a reduction in symptoms, particularly malodour. Of the remaining 12, six reported that their symptoms had reduced from a rating score of 6 to 0. One patient said, 'I feel and smell like a woman again; it makes me feel so much better.'	The reports of patients, carers and staff suggested that when NEOC is applied topically under a secondary dressing, it provides relief of some/all symptoms associated with FMWs with no documented adverse reactions and 100% user acceptability. These results suggest a promising potential product for management of FMWs.

REFERENCES

Bensouilah. J, and Buck. P, (2006) *Aromadermatology: Aromatherapy in the Treatment and Care of Common Skin Conditions.* Oxford: Radcliffe Publishing Ltd.

Bradley, B.F., Starkley, N. J., Brown, S. L., Lea, R.W. (2007) 'The effect of prolonged rose odour inhalation in two animal models of anxiety.' *Physiology and Behavior 92,* 5, 931–938.

Corner, J. (2008) 'Working with Difficult Symptoms.' In S. Payne, J. Seymour, and C. Ingleton (eds) *Palliative Care Nursing: Principles and Evidence for Practice.* 2nd edition. England: Open University Press.

da Costa Santos, C.M., de Mattos P.CA., Nobre, M.R. (2010) 'A systematic review of topical treatments to control the odour of malignant fungating wounds.' *Journal of Pain Symptom Management 39,* 6, 1065–1076.

Fleck, C.A. (2006) 'Palliative dilemmas: wound odour.' *Wound Care Canada 4,* 3, 10–13.

Gethin, G., Grocott, P., Probst, S., Clarke, E. (2014) 'Current practice in the management of wound odour: an international survey.' *International Journal of Nursing Studies 51,* 6, 865–874.

Georges J., Grypdonck M., Dierckx de Casterle, B. (2002) 'Being a palliative care nurse in an academic hospital: a qualitative study about nurses' perception of palliative care nursing.' *Journal of Clinical Nursing 11,* 6, 785–793.

Grocott, P. (2007) 'Care of patients with fungating malignant wounds.' *Nursing Standard 21,* 24, 57–58.

Hawthorn, M. (2010) 'Caring for a patient with a fungating malignant lesion in a hospice setting: reflecting on practice.' *International Journal of Palliative Nursing 16,* 2, 70–76.

Kiecolt-Glaser, J.K., Graham, J.E., Malarkey, W.B., Porter, K., Lemeshow, S., Glaser, R. (2008) 'Olfactory influences on mood and autonomic endocrine, and immune function.' *Psychoneuroendocrinology 33,* 3, 328–339.

Lehrner, J. Marwinski, G. Lehr, S. Johren, P., Deecke, L. (2005) 'Ambient odours of orange and lavender reduce anxiety and improve mood in a dental office.' Physiology and Behavior 86, 1–2, 92–95.

Low, W.L., Martin, C., Hill, D.J., Kenward, M.A. (2011)'Antimicrobial efficacy of silver ions in combination with tea tree oil against Pseudomonas aeruginosa, Staphylococcus aureus and Candida albicans.' *International Journal of Antimicrobial Agents 37,* 2, 162–165.

Mehrez, A., Maycock, P., Stringer, J., Mackereth, P. (2015) 'Managing hospital malodours with essential oils.' *In Essence 13,* 4, 14–16.

Mercier, D. and Knevitt, A. (2005) 'Using topical aromatherapy for the management of fungating wounds in a palliative care unit.' *Journal of Wound Care 14,* 10, 497–498, 500–501.

Paul J.C. and Pieper B.A. (2008) 'Topical metronidazole for the treatment of wound odour: a review of the literature.' *Ostomy Wound Management 54,* 3, 18–27.

Probst, S., Arber, A., Trojan, A., Faithfull, S. (2012) 'Caring for a loved one with a malignant fungating wound.' *Support Care Cancer 20,* 3065–3070.

Probst, S., Arber, A., Faithfull, S. (2013) 'Malignant fungating wounds – the meaning of living in an unbounded body.' *European Journal of Oncology Nursing 17,* 1, 38–45.

Stringer, J., Donald, G., Knowles, R., Warn, P. (2014) 'The symptom management of fungating malignant wounds using a novel essential oil cream.' *Wounds UK 10,* 3, 30–38.

Tavares, M. (2011) 'Integrating clinical aromatherapy in specialist palliative care.' Published by Marianne Tavares. Available at www.clinicalaromapac.ca, accessed on 12 November 2015.

Warnke, P.H., Becker, S.T., Podschun, R., Sivananthian, S. *et al.* (2009) 'The battle against multi-resistant strains: renaissance of antimicrobial essential oils as a promising force to fight hospital-acquired infection.' *Journal of Cranio-Maxollofacial Surgery 37,* 7, 392–397.

Warnke, P.H., Terheyden H., Açil Y., Springer I.N. *et al.* (2004) 'Tumour smell reduction with antibacterial essential oils.' *Cancer 100,* 4, 879–880.

Warnke, P.H., Sherry, E., Russo, P.A., Sprengel, M. *et al.* (2005) 'Antibacterial essential oils reduce tumour smell and inflammation in cancer patients.' *Journal of Clinical Oncology 23,* 7, 1588–1589.

Warnke, P.H., Sherry, E., Russo, P.A., Açil, Y. *et al.* (2006) 'Antibacterial essential oils in malodorous cancer patients: clinical observations in 30 patients.' *Phytomedicine 13,* 7, 463–467.

Chapter 10

PROGRESSIVE MUSCLE RELAXATION

Dr Peter A. Mackereth and Ann Carter

KEY WORDS
progressive muscle relaxation, stress, anxiety,
research, relaxation groups

INTRODUCTION

Two approaches that we have found useful in helping patients and carers to relax and to promote calm are progressive muscle relaxation (PMR), and guided imagery, which is covered in Chapter 11. This chapter aims to develop your understanding of the background to PMR and its potential use in one-on-one and group situations. We have included a sample script, which you can adapt to your own style and purpose for using PMR; the second part of the chapter covers some important aspects of setting up a relaxation group.

THE ORIGINS OF PMR

In 1905, Edmund Jacobson, the originator of the progressive muscle relaxation training, noticed that when students were deeply relaxed, they did not demonstrate an obvious startle response to a sudden noise. It was this observation that formed the origin of his life's work (Jacobson 1977). He developed a lengthy and meticulous technique that focused on an individual being in touch with the muscular system and learning how to control the levels of tension in the muscles. Jacobson's method was designed so that an 'indivdual' would reach a level of competence, where he/she would be able to unconsciously be aware of unwanted tension and would be able to release it. Others have adapted and shortened the process, principally Joseph Wolpe, a South African psychiatrist. Due to Wolpe's work, the technique became known as 'abbreviated progressive muscle relaxation training', which is now usually referred to as progressive muscle relaxation or PMR (Wolpe 1958). This adaptation includes a controlled tension-release cycle (e.g. taking the shoulders upwards towards the ears, acknowledging the tension and then releasing it in a controlled manner). The process is combined with paying attention to breathing (see Chapter 13).

SO HOW DOES THE PRACTICE OF PMR HELP TO CONTROL STRESS?

The sympathetic division of the autonomic nervous system (ANS) is associated with the 'fight-flight' response; it mobilizes the body in an emergency and in stressful circumstances. Patients are often familiar with the concept that a response to a stressful situation is triggered by the production of adrenaline or noradrenaline (Hucklebridge and Clow 2002). They may be less aware that as heart rate and blood pressure increase, muscle tension also increases as the body prepares to fight or flight. Additionally, patients may also be less familiar with the physiological reaction, that along with the response to a stressor, cortisol is released, which mobilizes sugars from the liver and inhibits the immune response. They may not fully understand that the stress response occurs when 'danger or a threat' may not be present in reality; it may be imagined, and the body reacts to the thoughts as if the 'stressor' were real.

We have found it useful to be able to explain the stress response to patients clearly and succinctly. When patients realize that the stress response is a natural process, and it is something we can all experience, they are often reassured that it is a 'common response'.

Freeman (2001) argues that PMR techniques blunt sympathetic arousal by training an individual to reduce oxygen requirements. This is achieved by the repetitive release of muscle tension combined with a slowing of breathing rates, making PMR a useful therapeutic intervention for panic, phobias and anxiety states. Stefano *et al.* (1996) have acknowledged that repetition of the tightening and relaxation of muscles is crucial to the relaxation response. They also maintain that belief or trust in the process may influence expected outcomes and can help to regulate immunological function through cognitive and neurological processes. Benson (1996) has described this sense of improved 'wellbeing' which is associated with the relaxation response as 'remembered wellness'; he has attributed this pleasant state to memories of nurturance and maternal attachment. Remembered wellness is key to utilizing PMR as a resource to support resilience (see Chapter 2).

HELPING PATIENTS TO LEARN PMR

PMR is a learned skill, which can be practised in a variety of situations, for example waiting rooms, before or during a procedure, or to promote sleep (Mackereth and Tomlinson 2010). Before undertaking a PMR session with an individual, it is essential that a case history is taken; PMR is a therapeutic intervention. The patient must be aware of the processes involved and the potential benefits. It is also essential to avoid using relaxation skills when the receiver has an altered state of reality and is unable to consent, is under the influence of drugs, (including alcohol) or where the individual doesn't want to participate.

PMR can be offered either in a single session by a suitably trained therapist or through a series of 'training' sessions, preferably in a quiet space. A major advantage of the physicality of the technique gives the patient something on which to direct his/her attention in less than ideal conditions, such as noisy environments. Anecdotal feedback suggests that patients like the process; they feel that they can refocus their minds through carrying out the tension/relaxation cycles which are characteristic of PMR. Even if it is not convenient to actively carry out the physical movements, patients tell us that just thinking of doing the actions involved can still be a helpful technique.

The therapist needs to ensure that the patient is lying down or sitting in a comfortable chair. The use of pillows is particularly helpful to support posture, limbs and joints, and a blanket needs to be available for warmth and security. Mobile telephones and pagers need to be turned off and a request made for 'no interruptions' during the training session (although a perfectly quiet environment in clinical setting cannot be guaranteed!).

'Squeezy balls' are a useful addition in helping patients learn the basic neuro-muscular skills implicit in PMR. By squeezing and relaxing the spongy balls, the motion involved in the tension/relaxation cycle can be reinforced. Patients can take the 'balls' away with them to assist practice. 'Balls' come in a variety of additional forms – animals, footballs, globes, cars and stars (see Figure 10.1). They can have varying resistances so they can be used to help people who have arthritis in their hands. 'Squeezy balls' are particularly helpful as their use increases the focus for the process and, where appropriate, they can be used to introduce gentle humour.

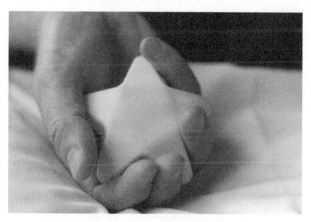

Figure 10.1: A 'star' example of a 'squeezy ball'

Ideally, a cycle of tension/relaxation is carried out with each muscle group an optimum of four times. Depending on the time available, and the physical condition of the patient, the number of cycles for each muscle group can be reduced. For comfort, we suggest that it is helpful for the patient to loosen a tight belt and to remove shoes. He/she may need to wrap him or herself in a blanket – either for security or for warmth. Sometimes, body temperature can drop during relaxation due to a slowing of the metabolic rate.

A sample script for using PMR is suggested below. Some therapists like to use the approach as described, and include a 'settling down' introduction. Other therapists like to begin straight away with the cycle of tension and relaxation, often starting with the feet. The following is intended as a guide and it is important that therapists create their own style of delivery.

A PMR sample script

I would like to invite you to become aware of different parts of your body – your feet, your calves, your thighs... (and then the therapists goes through all the parts of the body including the parts of the face, creating body awareness).

Then you may like to invite the individual to become aware of their breathing...by saying:

And now, it may be helpful to become aware of your breathing...and you may have already noticed that you are beginning to breathe a little more slowly than you were a few moments ago...and you may like to think to yourself, I am peaceful, I am calm, I am relaxed...or any words that mean the same thing to you.

And now let's continue with relaxing our bodies...

First, we are going to start with our feet. Gently curl your toes, and as you do so breath in, and as you release the curl, breathe out.

And next – I would like you to tense and relax your calf muscles...so turn your toes upwards towards the ceiling, and breath in as you do so. Feel the tension in your calves...and then breathe out as you relax the tension.

Continuing upwards through your body, the next area to go to is your thighs. Pull your thighs together and breathe in as you do so...feel the tension on the inside of your thighs, and possibly in your buttocks...and then relax the tension as you breathe out.

The next area where we are going to work is your abdomen (or tummy). Take a breath in and, like a balloon filling up with air, let your tummy expand outwards...and then, as you breathe out, let your tummy relax...(like a balloon losing air) and then let your tummy return to a neutral position and easy breathing. (Sometimes patients may find it helpful to put a hand on the abdomen so they can feel the sensation of movement.)

And now we are going to your hands... Make a fist with your hands, breathing in as you do so, and then relax the tension as you breathe out.

Continuing up your body the next area is your arms... As you breathe in take your hands up to your shoulders, bending your arms at the elbows, feel the tension...and then breathe out as you release the tension.

And now, let's go to your back...and as you breath in, pull your shoulderblades together...and as your breathe out release the tension.

And the next place is your shoulders...take your shoulders up to your ears, breathing in as you do so... Feel the tension, and then slowly, as you breathe out become aware of your shoulders being lowered and the release of tension.

And, finally, let's go to your face and scrunch up the muscles of your face – just as you would if you were pulling a funny face… Breathe in as you do so and then, as you breathe out, relax the face muscles and feel the tension leaving your face.

(Some people dislike tightening up their face muscles as they may think they look 'funny'. A gentle self-massage of the face has been found to be relaxing and seems to be acceptable to most patients. Rather than stopping the relaxation session abruptly, a pleasant way to bring the session to a close is simply for the individual to just stroke down his/her arms, from the shoulders to the fingertips two or three times, using the opposite hand.)

When you arrive at the end of the session, break the relaxation state by saying something like:

And now we have reached the end of the relaxation, I would like you to come back and join me in the room where we began… You may like to wriggle your fingers and toes…and slowly open your eyes…take a look around the room, noticing the curtains, and the chairs, becoming aware of any objects and so on.

COMING BACK TO EVERYDAY ALERTNESS

To bring the patient back to everyday alertness, you will need to raise your voice in order to break the patient's relaxed state and to get his/her attention. You can also increase the speed of your speech. If the person remains in a relaxed state, repeat the instructions firmly and a little more loudly, and change your own body position, for example by standing up. You may have to go over to the person and use his/her name firmly or put your hand on the individual's shoulder to help him/her realize that the session has finished.

MAINTAINING AGREEMENTS

Towards the 'end of relaxation stage' you have the choice of bringing the patient back to 'everyday alertness' or leaving him/her to drift for 'one minute of clock time', to listen to some relaxing music, or to conclude the session with a few minutes of guided imagery. If you agree with the patient to have a space of one minute at the end of the relaxation for 'individual time', create trust by maintaining the agreement. Perception of time may distort during relaxation; it may seem to go faster or slower than an everyday awareness of time. If a person knows that the 'individual time' is only one minute, it isn't usually a problem. However, if you suddenly decide to extend the time to five minutes, without agreeing it with the patient beforehand, you put the patient in a position of uncertainty and possible confusion as you haven't kept to the initial agreement.

THE SKILFUL USE OF LANGUAGE

The addition of positive suggestions are a useful part of the relaxation session. Early on in the session, it is useful to include some of the following suggestions:

- *'...if you experience any mental chatter during this relaxation, you can give the thoughts permission to be present and acknowledged, and then, when you are ready, return your attention to the sound of my voice'.* (See Chapter 11.)

- *'...as you are practising PMR, it is helpful to become aware that the movements you are practising can help to reduce tension and improve wellbeing'.*

- *'Long after this session is over, you can continue to experience and reinforce any of the positive things you have felt and learnt today.'*

- *'During your sleep tonight....as you breathe out your body will continue to relax more and more deeply...this will help you make the most of your sleep – and on waking feel more refreshed and recuperated.'*

Some patients tell us that when the therapist is no longer speaking, the thoughts start to present themselves again and this spoils what has been achieved (see Chapter 11). Others will tell us that once they 'got into it' they didn't hear a word the therapist said, and they drifted off into their own world. Few people like complete silence, and, at least to start with, we have found it can be helpful to have music playing quietly in the background.

COMBINING PMR WITH A CONVENTIONAL BODY WORK TREATMENT

Carlson and Hoyle's (1993) review of PMR literature concluded that one-to-one instruction was more effective than group sessions and depending on the time available, complementary therapy treatments can be an ideal opportunity for patients to learn PMR. The technique can have a place as a precursor to another complementary therapy intervention, where the goal is to prepare the body to consciously receive touch. For example, a patient can be so tense that they cannot imagine gaining anything from massage. PMR can also be taught as a post-massage self-soothing technique when the patient has experienced a measure of calmness and pleasure in the body. He/she can take charge of noticing tension, exaggerating it with the in-breath and then letting go of it with the out-breath.

SUPPORTING A PMR SESSION WITH A CD

Sometimes a patient will ask for a CD to reinforce practice. A PMR training CD, recorded by the therapist, provides an opportunity to support a patient who wishes to practice PMR independently. A CD can support, but does not replace, initial one-to-one training; however, a CD can be individualized to include suggestions specific to a patient's needs. We recommend that the CD is recorded 'live' where possible, when the therapist is working with the patient. We acknowledge that the CD may not be 'perfect', but it will have the advantage of anchoring the one-to-one session with the therapist as a resource. Recording CDs separately can be very time-consuming and frustrating, especially when a therapist is trying to make a CD at home without professional recording equipment.

RELAXATION GROUPS

Closed and open groups

Informal feedback tells us that relaxation groups are very popular in a variety of supportive care settings. The following covers some of the pleasures and pitfalls of running groups and details some issues that may be overlooked. If you are new to this activity, or if the relaxation group is a new initiative, we suggest that you run some pilot sessions and review progress before the activity becomes a permanent event.

Broadly, two main approaches to groups may be identified – one that is 'closed' and one that is 'open'. A closed group may be facilitated where the aims are to help patients with a specific problem, such as anxiety or fatigue. These groups usually have a fixed time limit, for example one session weekly for four to six weeks. Group members may be referred by a healthcare professional and once membership is agreed the group is closed. There are usually ground rules incorporated into the group life, which are agreed by the group members and the group leader in the first session.

The description 'open' implies that there is no finite membership and patients (and carers) can attend as they wish. This sounds a very flexible facility as patients can access the 'drop-in' when needed. However, the strength of flexibility can also present challenges. The group leader does not know in advance how many individuals will arrive and how many therapists need to be present. Individuals may have varying expectations of the group activities and have unrealistic expectations. Often, the group activity incorporates a taster session of a complementary therapy (such as aromatherapy, massage or reflexology) in addition to the relaxation session. If you are running a drop-in, we suggest that the taster sessions of complementary therapies are carried out first, and the relaxation session starts at a set time. The emphasis in this chapter is on running the open group, often facilitated as a 'drop-in' activity.

Boundaries – do we need them?

Preparation is the key to a successful group intervention. It is important that potentially tricky processes are considered either beforehand, or resolved as they arise. Boundaries are still important with this type of group – sometimes people attend on a continual basis rather than for a few sessions. The group begins to fulfil a social need for some people; it can provide much-needed company in a pleasant environment, which makes it difficult for some people to leave, and for new people to join in, especially where space is limited. It may be necessary to consider boundaries for attendance (subject to review) and for individuals to be aware of the built-in 'review of progress' system in place.

The need for helpers

It is always essential to have one or more helpers who are committed to supporting the therapist as the group leader, rather than having a 'relaxation session and treatment'. However, if you do have to work in a room on your own, make sure that you know how to summon help if needed. Relaxation can enable 'stuck' emotions to surface and it is useful to have someone on hand to help in whatever way is required.

Leading the group session

When leading a relaxation session we have found it helpful to adopt a similar relaxation position to the group if they are sitting in chairs. This is the most likely position for relaxation; many patients find it difficult to get comfortable on the floor, and they may find it difficult to get up at the end of the session. If group members are lying down, or if they are using a recliner, sit on a chair where you can see everyone.

We suggest that as you travel through the PMR process, you do the different actions involved in PMR yourself, with your eyes open. This helps you to pace your actions and your own speech in time with the group. If someone doesn't understand what you are saying, they can open their eyes and follow the actions from observation, rather than the verbal instructions. (This also applies to one-to-one teaching situations.)

We don't think it helps to walk around the room unless someone is having difficulty and needs attention. It can be disconcerting if your voice keeps coming from different places. If people are lying down, some people may feel you are going to tread on them. Keep your eyes open, whatever the situation, as you need to monitor what is happening.

Keep your feet firmly on the ground so that you remain grounded, and if you feel yourself getting sleepy, change your body position. You may also need to have water available for yourself (and for members of the group).

It is helpful if the area can be quiet, but, in reality, this is not always possible. So long as you seem confident, acknowledging new noises rather then pretending that they are not there, most intrusions can be dealt with. When disturbances arise it is usually best to acknowledge them and integrate awareness of the noise into the session.

Reassuring participants

When beginning the PMR session, the therapist leading the group may like to 'set the scene' by stressing a number of points to the group (or individual):

- Everyone works at his or her own level; you can sit and watch if you wish.

- If you want to keep your eyes open that is OK. It can be helpful to focus on some detail in the room such as the edge of a door or a window, or a pattern if the room is carpeted.

- Look after your own levels of comfort – tell us if you need something before we start or raise your hand during the session.

- If you need to cough, please do – it's unlikely anyone will notice! They will be too busy doing their own thing. There is plenty of water to help.

- Rumbly tums are welcome – it shows that relaxation is taking place.

- When you 're-enter' at the end of the session, you may want to open and close your eyes slowly two or three times before you fully return to alertness.

- There are no mistakes, only learning.

Leaflets containing information can be helpful for newcomers (and publicity), although it is not always possible for patients to access the information before they attend for the first time.

Use open, non-directive language

Keep the language you use 'open' so that you are not prescriptive. The scripts and suggestions in this chapter (and Chapters 11 and 12) give some useful examples. Some words and scenarios may have more significance for others rather than for you; it is important to 'suggest' or 'invite' group members to carry out the movement involved in PMR, rather than giving the instruction in a directive manner.

Challenges that can arise

As stated above, it is not appropriate for the leader to detach from the group by closing his/her eyes. Stay alert during the sessions as group members are in an altered state (and you may be too!). During the session the following could happen:

- someone is unable to join in and feels isolated
- coughing
- crying
- feeling unsafe
- panic/hyperventilation
- nodding off and becoming unsafe on a chair if sitting up
- snoring
- mobile phones ringing.

What does the lead therapist do if any of these things happen? Participants will expect you to take charge of unexpected situations. It the incident is resolvable without disturbing the group, verbally acknowledge that it is happening, Supposing someone was crying and wanted to leave the group room – you could say something like, 'I would like you to continue with the movement we started, I am just going to open the door so that Mary can take Sarah into a side room' and sit down and carry on. This is really when you need a helper who will take action for you. You can't continue with a relaxation session and support a distressed patient at the same time.

Most people will continue with the session as long as you let people know that you are in charge. Obviously, if it is impossible to carry on, bring the group back to the room slowly and confidently so that they keep their confidence in you.

Ending the session

At the end of the session, make sure that everyone is fully alert. Change the pace and volume of your speech so they know something different is happening. If someone does take a little longer to come round, use his/her name and ask the individual to open his/ her eyes so that he/she makes good eye contact with you. Invite a change in body posture, which is a good way to interrupt an altered state.

SUMMARY

This chapter has explored some of the principles on which PMR is based and has detailed some of the ways of carrying out this therapeutic approach for individuals and groups. A draft of a script for conducting a PMR session has been suggested, together with some ideas for running drop-in relaxation sessions. We have found PMR to be a most useful and enjoyable tool for therapists to offer and for patients to receive.

REFERENCES

Benson, H. (1996) *Timeless Healing: The Power of Biology and Belief.* New York: Scribner.

Carlson, C.R. and Hoyle, R.H. (1993) 'Efficacy of abbreviated muscle relaxation training: a quantitative review of behavioral medicine research.' *Journal of Consulting and Clinical Psychology 61,* 6, 1059–1067.

Freeman, L.W. (2001) 'Research on Mind-body Effects.' In L.E. Freeman, and G. Lawless (eds) *Complementary and Alternative Medicine: A Research Based Approach.* London: Mosby.

Hucklebridge, F. and Clow, A. (2002) 'Neuroimmune Relationship in Perspective.' In A. Clow and F. Hucklebridge (eds) *Neurobiology of the Immune System.* London: Academic Press.

Jacobson, E. (1977) 'The origins and development of progressive relaxation.' *Journal of Behavior Therapy and Experimental Psychiatry 8,* 2, 119–123.

Karagozoglu, S. Tekyasar, F. and Yilmaz, F. A. (2013) 'Effects of music therapy and guided visual imagery on chemotherapy-induced anxiety and nausea-vomiting.' *Journal of Clinical Nursing 22,* 39–50.

Mackereth, P. and Tomlinson L. (2010) 'Progressive Muscle Relaxation: A Remarkable Tool for Therapists and Patients.' In A. Cawthorn and P. Mackereth (eds) *Integrative Hypnotherapy: Complementary Approaches in Clinical Care.* London: Elsevier.

Stefano, G.B., Scharrer, B., Smith, E.M., Hughes, T.K. *et al.* (1996) Opioid and opiate immunoregulatory processes. *Critical Reviews in Immunology 16,* 2, 109–144.

Wolpe, J. (1958) *Psychotherapy by Reciprocal Inhibition.* Stanford, CA: Stanford University Press.

Chapter 11

GUIDED IMAGERY
Ann Carter and Dr Peter A. Mackereth

KEY WORDS
guided imagery, visualization, sensory language, relaxation, themes

INTRODUCTION

Guided imagery (GI), sometimes referred to as visualization or creative imagery, is frequently used in cancer care as a process to help patients access a state of relaxation. It may be used either as a single intervention or combined with other therapeutic approaches. First, this chapter provides a brief overview of some of the influences which have affected the development of GI since the 1980s. The advantages and disadvantages of using prepared scripts and patient-centred scenarios are discussed and the use of sensory language is explained and recommended. Some topics for themes that have been used on numerous occasions are suggested, and the content is illustrated by the use of case studies.

THE DEVELOPMENT OF GUIDED IMAGERY TECHNIQUES

Battino (2000) defined guided imagery as 'any internal work that you do that involves thoughts (uses the mind) and has a positive effect on health' (p.3). In this chapter, 'imagery' refers to a combination of visual, auditory, kinaesthetic and olfactory sensory experiences, rather than relying on the visual sense alone (Carter and Mackereth 2010). (The sense of taste can be included where it contributes to the activity.)

Possibly, one of the earliest techniques used in cancer care that included a mental/visual process was through the work of a radio-oncologist Carl Simonton. Simonton developed a multi-therapy approach that included cognitive-behavioural elements, relaxation exercises, guided imagery and meditation (Simonton, Simonton and Creighton 1980). Initially, the guided imagery component utilized a group approach, during which patients would 'visualize' cancer cells being destroyed by a 'stronger element' within the body. Later the technique was modified and the treatments were tailored to individuals (Battino 2000).

However, this and other approaches to GI have been developed by a range of experts drawn from physicians, cell biologists and psychologists (Achteberg 1985; Battino 2000; Borysenko, Dossey and Kolkmeier 1994; Leshan 1990). Further contributions have been made by the growing popularity of neuro-linguistic programming (NLP) and the therapeutic work carried out by psychologist and hypnotherapist Milton Erikson (Erikson and Rosen 1982). Additionally, the therapeutic approaches of mindfulness and meditation have made a significant contribution to the acceptability and practice of GI.

The processes involved in GI offer a practical and flexible therapeutic tool which can be used either on its own, or in conjunction with other therapeutic techniques, for example progressive muscle relaxation (PMR), massage, reflexology, HEARTS and other forms of body work. Ironically, where research into the effectiveness of GI has been carried out, it has often been in tandem with another therapeutic approach, thus making it difficult to ascertain the effectiveness of either therapeutic approach (Karagozoglu, Tekyasar and Figen 2013; Kwekkeboom and Bumpus 2008).

Initially, the focus for GI relied mainly on visualization so individuals would focus on what they could 'visual-eyes' or 'see' in the mind's eye. However, with the development of a variety of techniques from a range of disciplines, more resources are available to help patients to 'quieten the mind', so offering more choices to help patients achieve a potentially pleasant and relaxing experience.

EXPLAINING THE TECHNIQUES TO PATIENTS

Patients who are unfamiliar with the process may be concerned that they will not be able to 'empty their minds' or focus continually on 'only one thing' during the session. It is helpful for the therapist to simply explain the process; it is not necessary for an individual to have 'no thing' in their minds, or to focus on only one thing for the duration of the session, which may last from 5–15 minutes. A metaphorical approach which has been found to be useful in helping patients to understand the nature of thoughts and how they arise is outlined in Box 11.1.

Box 11.1: A simple explanation of the nature of thoughts and how they arise

The mind likes to produce thoughts, it is what it knows how to do. Sometimes when we are anxious or upset (or excited about something) the thoughts can seem to be overactive; we wish that we could slow them down or send them away altogether. The nature of our minds is to be active, and the thoughts which are present may have a physical effect on the body (Battino 2000; Dychtwald 1986).

There are easy-to-learn processes which will help to calm the mind and, through practice, the mind may be encouraged to become calmer. There is no need for anyone to empty their minds completely, or to focus on one thing for a period of time.

The basic principle is to encourage the mind to pay attention to a more peaceful, calm and enjoyable 'option' so it can find a more resourceful path of engagement. It is natural that everyday thoughts will enter into the mind from time to time and it is important that the patient does not begin a dialogue with these intrusions. The thoughts can be acknowledged and reassured that the individual will pay attention to them later, if necessary; they can be sent 'on holiday' or simply encouraged to pass through the mind. (A useful example is the way in which information passes along a 'news ticker' on television.) The patient returns to their 'enjoyable option'. If an individual starts a discussion with the thoughts, the thoughts may become even more active as they 'like to be noticed'. Borysenko (1997) suggests that it is the constant 'coming and going' of everyday thoughts alternating with a 'pleasant option' that brings about feelings of relaxation and the mind drifting into stillness.

Guided imagery is not the only therapeutic mental approach that discourages engagement with the thoughts; mindfulness and meditation adopt similar basic principles. During some GI sessions, the occurrence of everyday thoughts may be more intrusive, and sometimes the presence of thoughts may be calm. It is important that patients pay attention to the process, rather than deciding that the session was 'good or bad'. It may be helpful to remember that:

- Relaxing the mind is a process, not an event.

- The degree of mind relaxation achieved may vary from day to day.

- Practice does help. It is important not to judge success or failure – it is how it is!

Some patients will be motivated to practise the processes involved in GI, so that it becomes easily accessible and contributes to their resilience processes (see Chapter 2) Others will be content to come to a weekly group activity which they find beneficial (see Chapter 10).

SOURCING THE 'SCRIPT'

Some patients may have used commercial CDs to help with relaxation. Informal feedback tells us that if a patient dislikes the content, the accent, or the phrases used by the presenter, the content becomes irritating and the CD is not used after the first few listenings. It is important for the therapist to have an understanding of the range of approaches in making the most of 'scripts'. These approaches range from scripts which originate from the therapist's resources to those which have a patient-centred orientation.

A therapist-centred approach implies that the source for the 'script' is 'ready-made' to deliver to the patient. The words can be read directly from a book, or the script may have been adapted from a CD that the therapist likes or has experienced in another context. Sometimes, the therapist may 'personalize' a 'ready-made' script for individual patients (or for use with a group), although the patient(s) have had no direct input into the process. The choice of words and the suggested scenario is the therapist's choice. While being very convenient to use, prepared scripts may be counterproductive as they are incompatible with the individual(s) whom they are intended to help. Three such situations are outlined in the Box 11.2.

Box 11.2: Three examples of incompatible scripts

1. A therapist was taking a group session using a script which had been used on previous occasions. The script referred to a garden and contained a brief section where the group members were asked to 'visualize' themselves walking down seven steps. Elsie, whose legs were very edematous and bandaged, asked if this could be omitted; she said that 'walking down all those steps' was painful for her. The therapist, who was reading the script, forgot to omit the phrase, and Elsie winced as she counted every step described in the script. She felt she had to follow the instructions given exactly. The therapist did not look up from reading the words on the paper copy, so was unaware of Elsie's discomfort.

2. In discussion, Caroline told us that a phrase she didn't like was, 'Think of a white light entering your body through a hole in one of your feet.' She had sat through the 'relaxation' session wishing it would end, finding 'having a hole' in one of her feet quite distressing. Caroline did not say anything afterwards as she did not want to upset the therapist.

3. Jack had a good prognosis, but was still very anxious about his condition. His key worker suggested that learning 'visualization' would help him to relax. She suggested that Jack could 'visualize' himself walking on a beach at sunset, and offered a prepared script which reflected the elements of this scenario. Jack could not engage with this method; eventually he was referred to a therapist for massage as an alternative to the 'visualization'. Jack told the therapist that he did not like the content that was being suggested to him; he was a family man and while walking on the beach alone he missed his family. 'It was awfully lonely on that beach,' he said, 'I wanted my family with me.'

INVOLVING THE PATIENT

We have found that engaging a patient in constructing his/her own 'guided imagery option' a most worthwhile process. Involving a patient in this way promotes 'ownership' of the process for the patient and ensures that he/she is comfortable with the content and the language used. Using a patient-centred approach may also promote confidence in the individual to further develop his/her own resources (Carter and Mackereth 2010) (see Chapter 2).

When facilitating a patient-centred approach, we employ a framework based on sensory language to help construct a 'script' from the patient's experience. This process helps the patient to build a sensory 'image' of his/her choosing. Mainly, we use the three main senses: visual, auditory and kinaesthetic, and sometimes we include the olfactory sense. The gustatory sense doesn't always have a role to play, but it can be included where it has a contribution to make. Examples of sensory language are given below. This is not an exhaustive list, and there are many more sensory words that could be used.

Visual	Auditory	Kinaesthetic
see	sound	impact
focus	hear	feel
clear	whisper	touch
bright	rustle	tense
picture	crackle	rough
view	volume	cool
perspective	loud	warm
look	soft	relax
colour(s)	pitch	dance
hazy	muffled	fluffy
tinted	music	smooth
sparkle	harmony	velvet
shiny	whoosh	soft

STEPPING INTO SENSORY LANGUAGE

First, the therapist and patient agree a theme for the 'GI option'. The theme could be of a general nature such as a spring day, a seaside scene, or a favourite walk. (More examples of themes are given later in this chapter.) Other suggestions, which could draw directly on the patient's personal experience, could include an enjoyable experience, 'a time when you were calm', or 'a time when you felt confident'.

Once the theme is agreed, the therapist asks the patient to describe the experience in terms of what he/she can see, hear and feel, and/or smell. To avoid confusion, information about only one sense is requested at a time. As the patient describes his/her sensory experience related to an option of his/her choosing, the therapist will need to make some notes and then turn them into a script – this is normally by reading them back to the patient, rather like telling a story, and in a way that will facilitate relaxation.

This 'real-time' interaction, may seem a little daunting at first, but with a little practice, this approach can be an easy process which can be used anywhere, and at any time, without having to rely on a 'ready-made' script. It is the patient who already has the script and all we need to do is to help him/her to bring it into reality. Box 11.3 contains details of a brief script which was devised from notes that a therapist made when talking with a patient about a holiday in Spain. The patient had identified the holiday as a pleasant time in her life and was very eager to 're-enter' the experience.

As you read through the text, become aware of the sensory language used. This script includes the visual, auditory, kinaesthetic and olfactory senses. Interestingly, the sense used to access the scenario was olfaction, the patient having discussed the aroma of the oranges in the sunshine in some detail. We suggest that an introduction which helps to settle the patient can be added, and additional support can be accessed through the skilful use of music which has been agreed with the patient. There also needs to be a conclusion to the session, so that the patient knows the session has ended. Sometimes, a patient will go to sleep; rather than wake them up, we would usually tell a nurse that we have concluded the session and the patient is sleeping.

This approach could be used in conjunction with PMR, with a 'hands-on' therapy, as a resource for dealing with a procedure, or simply to provide a pleasant experience. Using patient-centred work of this nature is also particularly useful when working with aromasticks and HEARTS (see Chapters 8 and 12).

Box 11.3: An example of a script devised by a patient and using sensory language

And now, as you are sitting comfortably in your chair...begin to think of the aroma of the oranges...and I would like to invite you to let your mind drift back to the orange groves you were telling me about a few minutes ago...and as you find yourself walking through the rows of trees, you notice the dark green leaves of the citrus trees, decorated with the lovely ripe orange fruit... You may also become aware of the blue sky and the dry grass below your feet.

And...become aware of how lovely and quiet and peaceful it is, the quietness of the orange grove creating calm and tranquility, which you find yourself enjoying...

And as you experience the calm and tranquility of this place, notice how pleasantly warm the day is...becoming aware of a gentle breeze wafting over your face...increasing your awareness of the dryness of the ground underneath your sandals...and how good it feels to have the warmth of the sun shining on your shoulders... And now I would like to invite you to put this pleasant feeling you are experiencing somewhere in your body...where you can access it again...just by allowing your mind to drift back to this very pleasant time.

To illustrate how flexible this approach can be, a case history regarding the use of patient-centred guided imagery is given in Case study 11.1.

Case study 11.1: An opportunistic intervention in outpatients

Martin was awaiting treatment for a throat cancer. By chance he met the therapist who would be supporting him in the outpatients' department. The therapist outlined the complementary therapies she could offer and Martin asked if the therapist could do something 'there and then' so he could find out 'what relaxation was like'. Luckily, a room was available for half an hour. The therapist took some details relating to safety before asking Martin what he enjoyed before the cancer was diagnosed. Martin chose his garden, and admitted that since the diagnosis he had hardly given it a thought. The therapist helped Martin to build an image of his garden in terms of sight, sound, textures and aromas. Martin eagerly engaged with the progress, and as he talked he became more animated and smiling. At the end of the session, which took about 15 minutes, Martin was visibly more relaxed and had more colour in his face.

The next morning, Martin phoned to say that he had slept really well; for the first time in weeks he hadn't experienced nightmares about the treatment.

Some therapists have expressed concern that if a patient is involved in devising a personal script, they will become emotional and this could be counterproductive. We always ask patients to choose something that they are comfortable to work with, and very often, everyday things are chosen. Do remember that when an individual enters a state of relaxation, whether through a physical therapy, PMR or guided imagery, emotions may surface and sensitive processing can help them to feel calmer once a release has occurred.

USING PATIENT-CENTRED APPROACHES WITH GROUPS

This patient-centred method of devising a guided imagery session could be suitable for a group that meets regularly and where group members know and trust each other. It is more difficult to use where the membership of a group changes each week, such as in a drop-in activity. In this situation, the group members are unlikely to have built up trust with each other and may be apprehensive about 'saying the wrong thing', especially if it is the first time in attendence.

THE ROLE OF A PREPARED SCRIPT

There will always be a place for a prepared script, for example where a patient is finding it difficult to think of a scenario which he/she finds acceptable, or where the individual would feel more comfortable to receive a script that has been used to help other people (where it has been 'tried and tested'). In such situations, it is helpful if the therapist has something 'in mind' which he/she is familiar with and can easily recall. Where therapists are devising their own scripts, it is still useful to use a sensory language framework. It is important to offer choice and to be aware that some people cannot access the visual sense in their thoughts, and others may prefer to think in words

(Knight 2002, first published 1995). Some patients may prefer to receive more direct sensory experiences, such as massage, HEARTS and reflexology; however, they may like to access some imagery to enhance the physical therapy.

SUGGESTIONS FOR GUIDED IMAGERY SESSIONS

The following suggestions have all been used with groups and individuals either as a prepared script, or as prompts for patient-centred work. (Please note, this is not a finite list. There are many more options.)

- A visit to the countryside, the seaside, mountains, or a place of choice – create a pleasant experience around the visit.

- Think of a colour which represents relaxation to you, coming in through your body and replacing tension, leaving you calm and relaxed.

- Explore the seasons: spring, summer, autumn and winter, either at the beginning of the season (on the equinox) or thinking of the season that is coming next.

- Devise some imagery suggested by some aromas/essential oils, for example vetivert and bonfire night, cinnamon or orange for Christmas aromas.

- Go for a walk through the colours of a rainbow.

- A scenario from a good holiday.

- A memorable event, such as a wedding, a graduation, passing your driving test.

- A walk, somewhere that is locally familiar, or taking a dog for a walk.

- If you are worried about something, and your mind is overactive, put each unwanted thought into a bubble and let it float off into the atmosphere – so far away, it is out of sight and out of mind. You might want to replace it with something that represents confidence (or a positive resource) entering the body.

- Think of a treasure chest in which you can place and store resourceful memories, for example the best compliment you ever had, an achievement, something you are proud of, something you are committed to.

- Count backwards from 100, but if you lose the sequence you can go back to the beginning and start again.

- Think of a word you like and repeat it so it becomes similar to a mantra. Examples are 'peace' 'calm' or 'rest'. This principle may be applied to a poem, a prayer or a favourite proverb.

The last two ideas are useful options based on using the auditory sense on its own; this approach can be helpful where patients can't or don't wish to use their other senses. An example of its benefits is given in Case study 11.2.

Case study 11.2 Using the auditory sense

Joan was very motivated to learn a relaxation skill through using GI. However, she found that she couldn't access the scenarios that were suggested to her. She also admitted that she found seeing 'pictures' difficult. Finding that Joan liked to 'play with numbers' a second therapist suggested that Joan could try an auditory 'option' where she would start at one hundred and count backwards. If she lost the sequence, or the thoughts intruded, she had to go back to the beginning and start again. Joan really liked this approach. It was mechanistic and she could access numbers very easily. A further advantage was that she no longer felt a failure in not being able to engage with what the therapist had suggested.

We suggest that imagery sessions don't need to last for a long time to be effective, depending on the aim of the intervention. Battino (2000) recommends 15–20 minutes; interestingly, Achterberg (1985) found that people reached their maximum state of relaxation between 8 and 12 minutes and extending the time did not deepen the state of relaxation. In the context in which we work, we have found that 5–15 minutes can be sufficient time to provide a pleasant experience, for the patient to be engaged in 'a reverie' and to feel comfortable in one position. Our average length for including imagery after a PMR session is between five and eight minutes.

SUMMARY

We have found that helping patients to experience guided imagery has been a very useful process for both patient and therapist. When the patient is involved in creating the process, the options are limitless. The framework of using sensory language is a useful tool for therapists; they can help someone in an informal, opportunistic situation as well as using this framework for creating prepared scripts.

REFERENCES

Achterberg, J. (1985) *Imagery in Healing: Shamanism and Modern Medicine.* Boston: New Science Library.

Battino, R. (2000) *Guided Imagery and Other Approaches to Healing.* Camarthen: Crown House Publishing Ltd.

Borysenko, J., Dossey, B.M., Kolkmeier, L. (1994) *Rituals of Healing: Using Imagery for Health and Wellness.* New York: Bantam Books.

Borysenko, J. (1997) *Minding the Body, Mending the Mind.* New York: Bantam Books.

Carter, A. and Mackereth, P. (2010) 'Recognizing and Integrating "Hypnotic Trance" within Touch Therapy Work.' In A. Cawthorn, and P. Mackereth (eds) *Integrative Hypnotherapy: Complementary Approaches in Cancer Care.* London: Elsevier.

Dychtwald, K. (1986) *Bodymind.* New York: Penguin Putman.

Erikson, H.M. and Rosen S. (1982) *My Voice Will Go With You: The Teaching Tales of Milton H. Erickson.* New York: Norton.

Knight. S. (2002) *NLP at Work.* London: Nicholas Brearly Publishing.

Kwekkeboom K.L. and Bumpus, H. (2008) 'Patients' perceptions of the effectiveness of guided imagery and progressive muscle relaxation interventions used for cancer pain.' *Complementary Therapies in Clinical Practice 14*, 3, 185–194.

Leshan, L. (1990) *Cancer as a Turning Point.* New York: Plume.

Simonton, O. C., Simonton, S., Creighton, J. (1980) *Getting Well Again.* New York: Bantam Books.

Chapter 12

THE HEARTS PROCESS

Ann Carter

KEY WORDS

skin, sensory stimulation, bedclothes, relaxation, resilience, aromas

INTRODUCTION

HEARTS is an acronym for a group of therapeutic processes that support and strengthen patients with a variety of concerns and symptoms, so enhancing resilience (see Chapter 2). The acronym has been devised from the following components, the first letters of which make up the acronym:

Hands-on

Empathy

Aromas

Relaxation

Textures

Sound.

The HEARTS Process involves combining the different components to enable patients to achieve a relaxed, calm state quickly and easily. A HEARTS treatment can be effective in just a few minutes; alternatively, it can be included at any time during a conventional treatment involving massage, reflexology or guided imagery. Often referred to in the shortened form, 'HEARTS', the process always includes Hands-on physical contact, Empathy and the use of Textures (a patient is always covered during a treatment). The use of Aromas and Sound (either through the use of the human voice or music) are optional; either component can be used to enhance the process, or to facilitate

Relaxation when the patient may be finding it challenging to achieve this state.

This chapter explores the rationale for each component and how the process can be applied in a variety of settings. Case studies are used to describe some of the practical applications and the benefits.

BACKGROUND

In the early stages of working with patients in a supportive cancer care setting, the author came to the realization that many of the aromatherapy and massage techniques needed to be adapted for people experiencing different stages of cancer. Situations involving massage treatments which were particularly challenging for complementary therapists incuded:

- poor muscle tone

- cachexia

- friable/delicate skin

- poor absorption of a lubricant

- advanced metastatic spread

- mobility problems/positioning of patient.

It became clear that other approaches were needed, especially those which had the flexibility to be used wherever the patient was, whatever his/her condition and the time available. The question considered was, 'What other approaches could a therapist use that would promote a state of calm and relaxation quickly and easily?' Inspiration for the approach came from the lines of the poem by Tennyson:

But O! for the touch of a vanished hand,
And the sound of a voice that is still.

(Autton 1989, p.108)

IDENTIFYING WHAT WORKS

Through patient feedback and therapist experience, a variety of techniques were included when designing bespoke treatments for individuals. These techniques were those which patients found particularly welcoming, easy to receive and relaxing. They were simple, uncomplicated and were drawn from a variety of therapies. All of them could be adapted so complementary therapists, healthcare professionals and carers could use them. The first experience with a patient using the 'Hands-on' component of HEARTS is described in Case study 12.1.

Case study 12.1: Working through textures

George had a history of lung cancer. He was referred to the therapist for six one-hour sessions of aromatherapy massage. Although he was seemingly 'well', it was only when George attempted to remove his shirt it was clear that his co-ordination was poor and this task was difficult. He had requested a back massage and wanted to lie prone on the couch; in spite of the use of several pillows for support, George was uncomfortable. The oil was not absorbed into his skin and the therapist was concerned that a conventional aromatherapy massage approach was not the best use of time – although George insisted he had enjoyed the session.

The following week, the therapist suggested that George remain clothed. He remained seated and was supported by pillows as he leaned against the couch. The therapist covered him with a warm bath sheet on which she placed two drops of lavender essential oil (which George had previously requested). She used stroking movements through the texture of the bath sheet on George's back and arms, pausing to do some gentle holding techniques where she felt intuitively it would be beneficial. After five minutes George said, 'Aye, that's grand' and the therapist felt confident that this was a more productive approach and a better use of time.

WORKING WITH THE SENSORY SYSTEM OF THE SKIN

The skin is a remarkable organ, often reduced to a clinical diagram in a book; the accompanying text describes the functions of the skin and the diagram shows its structure. Neither the text nor the diagram fully explains the amazing properties of skin in terms of being a transmitter of sensory experience. Some properties of the skin, which demonstrate its potential role as a 'sensory canvas', are outlined by Montagu:

The surface area of the skin has an enormous number of sensory receptors receiving stimuli of heat, cold, touch, pressure and pain. A piece of skin about the size of a small coin contains more than 3 million cells, 110–340 sweat glands, 50 nerve endings and 3 feet of blood vessels. It is estimated that there are some 50 receptors per 100 square millimeters, a total of 640,000 sensory receptors... The number of sensory fibres entering the spinal cord by the posterior roots is well over half a million. The only organs with a larger surface area are the gastrointestinal tract and the alveoli in the lungs. The surface area of the skin is approximately 19 square feet in the average adult male, in whom it weighs 8 pounds, containing some 5 million sensory cells, the skin constitutes some 12 per cent of body weight. (1986, p.7, first published 1971)

With such a large sensory network, it is likely that skilful touch may be applied to small areas of the body for short amounts of time to promote a relaxation response. The sensory receptors are remarkable at detecting the minimum of sensory experiences. The smallest of changes in temperature, textures, and pressure can be distinguished. For example, while walking, a grain of sand can be detected in a shoe and a patient in his/her bed can detect a single biscuit crumb! An individual, with his/her eyes closed, can detect the differences between the textures of velvet, silk and cotton. The skin is sensitive enough to detect a gentle breeze or a minute change in temperature – although no physical contact has apparently taken place. This degree of sensitivity opens up a huge range of possibilities for working with an individual, in addition to the more conventional approaches to massage and other methods to body work.

Traditionally, massage tends to focus on releasing tension in muscles and increasing circulation through rubbing work (effleurage), squeezing, wringing and tapotement; to achieve its aim, this approach requires a lubricant. However, in the context of HEARTS, the skin is regarded as a 'sensory canvas' on which the hands, working as 'brushes', can 'paint their art'; the textures of clothes or fabric covers provide an interface between therapist and patient.

HANDS ON: THE 'LIBRARY OF STROKES'

To facilitate touching patients in a caring way, HEARTS uses the concept of a 'Library of Strokes' as a resource. This Library of Strokes may be defined as infinite ways of touching someone, which brings about either a calming or relaxing experience. The patient remains covered, and even in hot weather, being covered with a cool cotton sheet can offer a refreshing experience.

Anecdotally, feedback from patients and therapists suggests that the following 'strokes' offer an experience which both parties enjoy receiving and giving:

- Stroking movements along the body, or in circles, with the aim of creating relaxation using the palms of the hand. These movements are based on effleurage, but the texture of the fabric and the friction (which moving hands encounter) will not allow for heavy work. Maintaining a rhythm is the key, so the therapist avoids any pressure. (If there is too much pressure the fabric may wrinkle and the friction will be noticeable on the therapist's hands.)

- Finger brushing – for light work and pleasant surface sensations.

- Holding techniques – to promote a sense of quiet and calm.

- Gentle pressures and palming – for promoting a sense of security. (Palming is an ancient technique based on a major component from Thai massage and Shiatsu.)

- Breeze strokes using the hand(s) about one inch above the physical body – this approach is not concerned with chi, the person's aura or chanelling any form of healing energy. The movements seek to be non-invasive and create flow, sometimes warmth and even a sensation of gentle care around an area. They are a good way to finish off a treatment.

Working in twos – or more!

When using the principles on which the Library of Strokes is based, there are many situations where more than one therapist can work with a patient at a time (see Figure 12.1). This work can be pleasant to give and to receive for both the therapists and the patient. It can also be easy, and beneficial, to involve carers in using this approach; they can learn techniques for use at home or when a therapist is not present. Patients can also return selected approaches from the Library of Strokes to their carer(s), thus providing a two-way 'giving back' experience, so that patient does not feel that he/she is always the receiver. Sometimes, patients feel that care is always given in a one-way direction and they may feel that loved ones are 'missing out' (see Chapter 14). An example of a situation involving a carer is given in Case study 12.2.

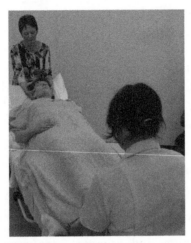

Figure 12.1: Paired: it is easy for two therapists to work together – a carer can easily be involved

Case study 12.2: Using HEARTS to help support both a patient and a carer

The therapist was invited to find out how she could help John and Mary. John had received bad news and the couple looked very downcast. They asked the therapist if there was something they could do for each other, as John did not want to be 'having all the attention'. The therapist noticed how pale John was and invited him to get back into bed. With John's permission, she covered one arm with a towel, and said, 'Now all you need to do is to follow my fingers as they stroke from your shoulder down through your elbow...down through your forearm...and down through your hands and then into your fingers.' The therapist continued repeating the sentence (in slightly different ways) and John closed his eyes. Mary was invited to join in with the stroking on the other side of the bed, following what the therapist was doing. The colour started to come back into John's face very quickly and after five minutes he said, 'Do you know, I feel so much better, more like a cloud has lifted.' The therapist helped the couple learn some different approaches, including a hand massage without oil. The couple established a routine giving and receiving some kind, well-intentioned touch in the morning and evening throughout John's stay in the hospital.

Varying the 'strokes'

The 'strokes' described in the Library of Strokes are not an absolute in themselves. Each stroke can be varied by the speed the therapist uses, the pressure, the length of the stroke, the area of the body covered, the rhythm, and the texture of the fabric through which the stroke is applied. (The use of textures will be covered later in the chapter.) The strokes used can be experienced and agreed by the patient before the session starts so that he/she 'knows what's coming' and can remain in control of the Hands-on work.

Factors that may influence the ability to receive 'kind', well-intentioned touch

The degree to which a patient feels able to receive touch may depend on his/her 'touch history'. Patients are likely to have received different kinds of touch during their lives, some of which may not have been welcome. Physical touch may have been manipulative or conditional, or associated with violence and abuse. Importantly, in the cancer care context touch may also be linked with medical procedures and investigations; one or more of these past experiences may make a patient wary about what the therapist may be offering.

A major advantage of working through clothes and covers is to physically provide an 'interface' which can offer modesty and safety, without the intimacy of using a lubricant and working at the 'hand to skin' boundary. With aging, and with the inevitable loss of partners, friends, family members and pets, some individuals may well experience profound 'skin hunger' (Buckle 2003) and have a need for being touched with kindness, which is offered physically, emotionally and spiritually (see Chapter 15).

EMPATHY

Mitchell and Cormack (1998) suggest that empathy is an essential component of all therapeutic relationships and applies to all patient–therapist interactions. Often, 'empathy' is related to listening, verbal interactions and body language. In the context of HEARTS, empathy also manifests in the way the hands are used, and how the different components are interlinked. The ability to choose and apply each component in harmony with another helps to facilitate a synergistic effect. Therapists need to be aware of the emotional power of the hands to convey non-verbal messages of empathy and safety, as well as caring, and where appropriate, affection. We encourage all therapists to remember that hands can communicate very eloquently, when we are truly present with another person. For some patients who are not used to receiving kind, respectful and thoughtful touch, the initial contact alone may be enough to create an emotional response. HEARTS can offer a shared 'whole person' experience, which can create new 'sensory and skin memories' as a resource for now and the future (see Figure 12.2).

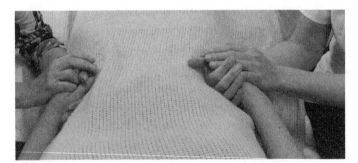

Figure 12.2: The hands are very eloquent, if only they are allowed to be

AROMAS

The aromas of essential oils can be can be used to generate olfactory pleasure, feelings of calm, wellbeing, relaxation, comfort – or whatever the aroma suggests to the individual. In recent times, the use ofaromasticks (aromatic inhalers) has enabled the pleasant experiences of complementary therapy treatments to be 'anchored', so the patient can reproduce the feelings of relaxation when 'sniffing the aroma' from the inhaler (Carter, Maycock and Mackereth 2011) (see Chapter 8). Not all therapists or healthcare professionals who use HEARTS are aromatherapists, and a qualified aromatherapist needs to prescribe a suitable essential oil or blend for the patient. However, most people have an aroma they associate with a positive memory; they can recall this memory without the physical aroma being present, for example aromas associated with bread-baking, holidays, flowers, gardens and the countryside. Recalling an aromatic memory can be a starting point for relaxation and has been found to be a useful resource for the therapist and patient. (Further suggestions for using this capability as a resource are given in Chapter 11.)

RELAXATION

This is the main aim of using The HEARTS Process. Achieving a state of relaxation, or a resourceful state of calm, is beneficial to patients, carers and healthcare professionals. Ryman (1995, p.3) has described relaxation as 'a state of consciousness characterized by feelings of peace, and release from tension, anxiety and fear'. When a patient enters a relaxed state it is more than 'doing nothing' and could be experienced as a 'reverie'. This state can be similar to the experience of floating into or emerging from sleep. Many patients become tolerant of living with stress and tension, unaware that the body has its own rebalancing capabilities, which can redress the less desirable state and promote a sense of calm.

TEXTURES

Textures of fabrics play an important role in HEARTS. Sanderson (1991) discusses the role that sensory stimulation plays in the rehabilitation of young adults with learning difficulties. Using this principle, and the knowledge that there are many body work therapies where the patient remains clothed, it was decided that rather than regarding dressing gowns, blankets and duvets as a hindrance, their textures could be used to enhance the sensory experience implicit in the Hands-on work. A patient can be covered with a warm towel, which can promote feelings of security, or he/she may be wrapped in a soft blanket, which offers memories of nurturing. For patients who are wary about too much intimacy where touch therapies are concerned, the extra 'layer' of cover can provide an interface which offers a sense of boundary.

Every time the therapist changes the texture through which he/she works, the patient will receive a different sensory experience, and the therapist can vary the Library of Strokes accordingly. Patients with limited co-ordination and/or those who have body image concerns do not have to undress. This principle of covering the patient, rather than asking them to remove clothing, is an important component of HEARTS.

SOUND

Frequently, when giving treatments, complementary therapists rely on music to promote an environment of relaxation. We live in a world of noise, often without choice. Silence is often a missing experience, which, when offered purposefully, can bring its own ambience, stillness and peace. The human voice can be a useful resource, especially when used together with well-intentioned touch. Many patients are very aware of 'mind chatter' and the use of the therapist's voice can help the patient to refocus on something more resourceful.

Utilizing the voice, its tone, pace and rhythm can be honed through practice and does not need to be continuous. It can be used at any stage in the treatment, adjusting the volume and the 'commentary' so it is seamless and flowing with the physical Hands-on touch.

Through working with patients, it has been found that touch, together with offering some easy verbal options for the mind, can guide people to enter a relaxed state more easily than when the Library of Strokes is used on its own. In HEARTS, the voice is used in conjunction with Hands-on work to make the most of sensory experience; the additional use of the voice should be agreed with the patient before the work begins. The advantage of using the voice is that it is a resource that a therapist has with him/her all the time. It is not always easy to arrange for music to be played on a busy and noisy ward at the precise time required.

One of the easiest ways of using the voice is to ask the patient to 'become aware' of different parts of the body, as the therapist places his/her hands on the area on which he/she is commenting. The therapist tells the patient where his/her hands are and asks the individual to become aware of the contact. It is suggested that this process is carried out in a logical sequence so the patient can recall the sequence, if required. A script is not required for this work; if the therapist is truly 'tuned in' to the patient, the patient's own body can be used to indicate the sequence to follow. For the therapist, the key is to maintain a natural conversational style as if this were an everyday occurrence, to use a slower speed of speech and to slightly lower the tone of the voice. It is also helpful for the patient to be able to voice any areas where he or she does not want to be touched before the treatment begins.

Some suggestions for using the voice to accompany the Library of Strokes are outlined below.

Diverting attention – using the kinaesthetic sense

Place your hands gently in an appropriate place such as the feet, hands or wrists. Bring the individual's awareness into your hands, for example, 'I would like to invite you to become aware of my hands resting on your feet...' and then you can work up the body, putting your hands on the 'landmarks'. The easy 'landmarks' are the feet, ankles, knees, outer thighs, upper hips, wrists, arms, hands, under the neck and head. You could say something like, '...and now become aware of my hands resting on your knees...and now take your attention to my hands resting on your hips – and notice that as you bring your awareness to the place where my hands are resting, that you may feel more relaxed...'

You can work through the 'landmarks' in this manner, commenting on where your hands are placed.

The ongoing commentary – the comfort journey through the body

Gently, hold the patient's feet, hands, wrists, knees or head – whichever is convenient and comfortable for both therapist and patient. Suggest that the person notices what it is like for him/her to have your hands in that position. Patients usually notice things like an experience of a sense of warmth, comfort and calm. Prompt if necessary, for example, if the patient says, 'It's nice', do offer them some suggestions that shift attention from a 'grateful' word to an embodied sensory experience, for example '...it might be warm...soothing or calming', delivered in a tone that reflects those offered words.

Then ask the patient to allow this pleasant feeling to travel round his/her body – you suggest where it is to go, keeping your 'instruction' in sequence. This is like a commentary – the significant areas are in front of you using the aforementioned 'landmarks'.

Using a relaxing, calming colour

Ask the patient to think of a colour that represents relaxation or calm – you don't need to know what it is. You can agree the entry point for the colour to enter the body before you start the session. With your hands in contact with the individual, ask him/her to bring the colour into the body and let it travel to different areas, using the 'landmarks' and tracking the movement of the colour, bringing with it a feeling of relaxation and calm, softening and relaxing tissues… visiting the various landmarks in sequence.

A variation is to ask what the individual needs at the time (see Case study 12.3). Think in terms of calm, peace, strength, humour – or whatever is important for the patient. There is no need for the patient to tell you exactly what he/she needs; some patients would be embarrassed to admit they need anything. When the person has thought of something, ask him/her to relate it to any colour that represents this state for him/her. Once again, you do not need to know what it is. As a therapist, the advantage of not knowing is that you cannot add your own experience of the colour. Our goal is not to impose any beliefs around colour – any colour(s) or none is good enough.

Then you make up a 'mini script', using the landmarks on the body as outlined above. You may need to reassure the patient that it is OK if the colour changes. An example of the use of colours is given in Case study 12.3.

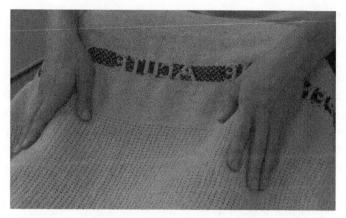

Figure 12.3: Making contact with one part of the body can be the start of a calming, relaxing session when the voice is used at the same time

Case study 12.3: Using a colour

Simon had been caring for his partner at home for some time and was finding the pressure overwhelming. He came for a complementary therapy treatment after having had a terrible argument. It was obvious that Simon was not in a good place, as he didn't want to talk about it. Once Simon was comfortable on the couch, the therapist suggested that he might like to think of what he needed 'right now' adding, 'and you don't need to tell me what you are thinking'. Simon nodded an acknowledgement that he had thought of something. The therapist asked Simon to link whatever he needed to a colour. With Simon covered with a blanket, the therapist used the 'landmarks' and invited Simon to take the colour round his body, taking with it whatever was needed 'right now'. After two or three minutes, the colour came back into Simon's face and his breathing became more relaxed. The therapist continued with the HEARTS treatment without speaking again. At the end of the 25-minute session Simon disclosed, without prompting, that what he wanted was 'strength' and had chosen the colour orange. When the therapist first began 'the script' he only experienced 'a pale lemony colour' but as the session continued the yellow became stronger and brighter. As he left, Simon said, 'I feel more able to cope with the situation at home now' (see Chapter 2).

SUMMARY

The HEARTS Process is simple yet profound in its benefits. It strengths come from working with a combination of techniques to help calm and rebalance body and mind. A major advantage is that it can be used anywhere for short, or longer, periods of time and patients can remained clothed. Patients who may find relaxation challenging respond well to the combination of skilful touch and the human voice. It is also a relaxing experience for whoever is doing the giving. It is an approach that can be taught easily to health professionals, as well as therapists. Carers can also learn some of the approaches, and informal feedback suggests that they find it a beneficial and helpful process.

REFERENCES

Autton, N. (1989) 'The Care of the Aged, Dying and Bereaved.' In B. Autton *Touch: An Exploration.* London: Dartman, Longman and Todd.

Buckle, J. (2003) *Clinical Aromatherapy: Essential Oils in Practice.* New York: Churchill Livingstone.

Carter, A., Maycock, P., Mackereth, P. (2011) 'Aromasticks in clinical practice.' *In Essence 10,* 2, 16–19.

Montagu, A. (1986) *Touching: the Human Significance of Skin.* New York: Harper and Row.

Mitchell, A. and Cormack, M. (1998) *The Therapeutic Relationship in Complementary Health Care.* Edinburgh: Churchill Livingstone.

Ryman, L. (1995) 'Relaxation and Visualization.' In D. Rankin-Box (ed.) *The Nurses' Handbook of Complementary Therapies.* Edinburgh: Churchill Livingstone.

Sanderson, H., Harrison, J., Price., S. (1991) *Aromatherapy and Massage for People with Learning Difficulties.* Birmingham: Hands On Publishing.

Chapter 13

EASING THE BREATHING BODY

Dr Peter A. Mackereth, Paula Maycock and Lynne Tomlinson

KEY WORDS
breathlessness, anxiety, techniques, adaptations, imagery

INTRODUCTION

Most people will have experienced breathlessness (dyspnea) at some time in their lives. After pain, it is the second symptom experienced by many cancer patients, and is often difficult to manage in the advanced palliative stage. In this chapter, we share techniques, which can assist patients to ease breathing and assist with respiratory function and resilience through regular practice. The techniques can be provided singularly or as 'stackable resources' with benefits increased by combining techniques. These techniques can be combined with other treatments of aromatherapy, massage and relaxation therapies (and other forms of body work).

BACKGROUND

Breathlessness has both physical and non-physical aspects; like pain, it can be defined by what a patient says it is. For many, breathlessness is an unpleasant sensation of being unable to breathe easily or a feeling of 'not getting enough air'. In patients who are living with, or recovering from, cancer treatment, there may be more than one underlying physical reason for breathlessness. Aside from local disease, the patient may have inflammation, scar tissue from treatment, a chest infection or pneumonia. Ability to inflate the lungs may be compromised by past or recent surgical removal of lung tissue, fluid collection in the pleural space, ascites in the peritoneal cavity or the effects of medication on respiratory drive. It needs to be remembered that patients living with cancer, may have other co-morbidities affecting the exchange and transport of gases, such as anaemia, heart disease, or long-standing respiratory problems, for example asthma, chronic obstructive pulmonary disease and emphysema. Physical effort, the presence of infection, altered metabolism and surgical trauma all create an increase in the demand for oxygen by the tissues. The sensation of breathlessness can be modified by higher cortical experience, which can encompass memory of fear and anxiety. In addition, associated symptoms of wheezing, coughing, and difficulty with breathing when lying down can compromise sleep and so increase exhaustion and fatigue (Molassiotis *et al.* 2010).

Lung function and the ability to utilize oxygen may also be affected by environmental and lifestyle factors. At the top of this list is smoking, with 40 per cent of patients using tobacco and other smoked/inhaled substances at the time of diagnosis. Lung cancer is associated with smoking histories in 80–90 per cent of cases (Eriksen, Mackay and Ross 2012; Parkin, Boyd and Walker 2011). In addition, passive smoking and chewing tobacco and betel leaf are also known risks for cancers (Secretan *et al.* 2009). Obstruction of the upper airways through local tumours, with smoking and alcohol also known risk factors, may require formation of a tracheal stoma to facilitate breathing and expectoration.

Deterioration in respiratory function and oxygenation of the tissues, either acute or chronic, can significantly reduce physical activity. Without intervention and preventative work, patients can quickly spiral downwards in terms of respiratory muscle tone and strength and loss of confidence in coping with exertion (Booth, Silvester and Todd 2003). Emotional distress can increase muscle tension and holding, as if there were a threat in the room. Where fleeing or fighting is not possible, inhibited breathing can trigger a 'caught in the headlights' response and a sense of being overwhelmed. The body risks becoming held in postures linked to chronic patterns of breathing, which can also fix thinking and behaviour. Literally, the fear of exacerbating breathlessness blocks any new activity or social engagement outside routines, which are perceived to be manageable. Increased dependency, lack of support and/or a reluctance to depend on others can result in isolation and withdrawal from any interests, hobbies and activities that require any exertion. As a consequence, the patient can experience a vicious cycle of breathlessness, anxiety and inactivity, which can lead to reduced resilience and depression. Being continuously breathless, or experiencing episodes of acute breathlessness which can easily be triggered, can bring heightened attention to the anxiety and even catastrophic interpretations, the most common panic symptom being fear of imminent death (Tishelman *et al.* 2007). Family, friends and even health professionals may inadvertently exacerbate this state, by fostering dependency for fear that the breathless person worsens in front of them.

THE '3B PLAN' FOR EASING THE BREATHING BODY

We suggest the following model for therapists to utilize in their practice; the techniques described in this chapter can be used across the three scenarios outlined below.

1. Building respiratory resilience. The daily or more frequent use of techniques with the purpose of exercising the 'respiratory tree', which can encompass the whole body. This metaphor is useful to promote the idea of visualizing the amazing structure that supports and transports breath.

2. Being prepared for an event. The patient prepares techniques to use prior to a known stressor or planned activity involving physical exertion. Practice, and an understanding of respiratory function and/or physiology, will help to embed the techniques. There is time to comfortably rehearse, become confident with the techniques and for body and mind to become more aware and resilient.

3. Breaking the cycle. The stages are to de-escalate, regulate and then reflect. The therapist can be called to assist in a situation where a procedure or situation has triggered anxiety and distress. Patients are often open to interventions offered in these scenarios – the key is asking patients to notice how techniques (remember offering a choice is empowering) and even the offer of assistance from a therapist can de-escalate anxiety.

THE 'BREATHING' THERAPIST

A key foundation to working with breathlessness is to have both an understanding of the disease and treatment, and a basic understanding of respiratory physiology and anatomy. Working within a multidisciplinary team provides opportunities to understand the role of the physiotherapist, respiratory therapist and medical interventions. These could include the use of airways medication, humidified oxygen, positioning, methods of promoting expectoration of sputum and strategies to manage fatigue and to ease a troublesome cough.

Using some of the techniques in this chapter can help to build resilience into the patient's system. Remember, as a therapist, the act of demonstrating the techniques, can also be a helpful and calming workout for your own breathing body. At the outset, it is important to balance bringing attention to breathlessness (and related anxiety) with building capacity and resilience during a therapeutic treatment. Words related to breathing can be loaded in meaning and interpretation. Simply instructing patients to relax and breathe deeply may actually trigger distress, as we cannot assume they can do either or both. As a 'starter' to a therapy session, it can be helpful to invite curiosity about breathing (Ramponi 2012). For example, the patient could be invited to observe how his/her body feels over the space of four breaths during a treatment. We also suggest the following questions:

- When you breathe in and out, are you aware of any tension in your body?

- Can you shift your position during therapy so that you feel more comfortable as you breathe in and out?

- How do you use your belly and back muscles when you breathe in and out?

- Is there a potential to breathe out (or in) a bit more at the end of an out-breath or an in-breath?

(Therapists will benefit from trying out these observations and questions in relation to their own breathing patterns.)

MAKING THE MOST OF RESPIRATORY FUNCTION: SNIFFING AND HUFFING

By sharing anatomical and physiological knowledge with patients (and carers) it can help to engage them in the understanding of their own bodies and in using and practising the techniques. For example, a breath can be 'topped up' by sniffing within two seconds of an inhalation and before an exhalation. This relies on explaining to the patient that the lungs have elasticity; they can stretch with an increase in pressure. As a therapist, drawing the edges of your lungs on your own body, using a finger during inspiration and expiration can help patients visualize the movements and capacity in their own system. As inhaled gases move to fill the air sacs, airway pressure starts to move down a gradient, so there is potential to open the airways a little more. Sniffing on top of an inhalation can be like topping up an internal stretchable balloon. On breathing out, making a huffing sound from the base of the chest, while pulling the arms in together can support expiration of the airways; a useful image is that of a set of bellows. Using this method we can expire more after an exhalation, so allowing us to move in more air during the next inhalation. As an exercise, breathing in this way can build respiratory capacity.

USING THE BELLY AND BACK MUSCLES

As a therapist, you can bring the patient's (and carer's) attention to how amazing the belly and back muscles are in breathing and how their use can be enhanced. For example, using a bed table and pillows for support, invite the patient to lean forward onto the pillows. Starting between the scapulae, the therapist rests his/her hands lightly on the patient's back (see Figure 13.1). Without speaking, the therapist can lighten the touch moving with the patient's in breath – on the exhale, the therapist can lean gently and slowly into the body, which promotes emptying.

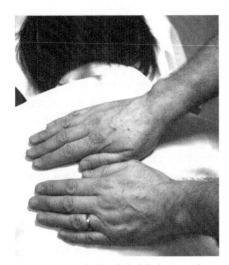

Figure 13.1: Resting the hands lightly between the scapulae

We call the process 'packing and emptying' and it can be repeated a further three times, the therapist's hands moving down the back, towards the buttocks. We also suggest a slight shaking or wobbling of the soft tissues at the end of the patient's exhalation. You may notice that as the patient 'lets go' of any tension, a ripple of movement may flow to other parts of the body; this is known as 'tensegrity', suggesting greater integration of the individual's underlying connective tissue (Hutson and Ellis 2006). This technique can raise awareness of how the wider body can become more engaged, and be a greater resource in breathing.

NOSTRIL FLARING AND AROMASTICKS

The simple technique of nostril flaring during inspiration can also bring awareness of how we can subtly begin the process of opening the airways. You can demonstrate this by putting your fingers either side of the nostrils and gently pulling the tissues in the direction of the ears so exaggerating this. Neuenschwander, Molto and Bianchi (2006) reported benefits for a group of patients living with breathlessness and advanced cancer; they used adhesive strips to facilitate nasal flaring. Nasal strips are available commercially as an aid to reduce snoring or for athletes in exercising. The addition of an aromastick to follow this technique can increase the opening of the nasal airway and add to the olfactory experience (see Chapter 8). Similarly, a chosen aromastick can also be stacked with other techniques, for example with sniffing and huffing.

PALM OPENING

This involves working with the wider body. You can invite the patient, if standing, to loosely hang their arms by his/her sides. Then ask the person to rotate the arms so the palms of the hand face fully forwards (palm opening); this will naturally open the chest on inhalation. If the patient is seated, a narrow pillow or bolster length can be placed behind his/her back; this will support the upper body and head and exaggerate the result. On expiration, the arms hang down with the palms turned to face backwards. You can suggest opening the knees during inspiration, and bringing the knees back together during expiration, thus making it a whole body exercise. Patients can be asked to repeat these movements three more times.

BREATHING BODY IMAGERY COMBINED WITH MASSAGE AND REFLEXOLOGY

Therapists can consider including visual words and metaphors in any therapeutic work; some patients may find this helpful depending on their own learning style. We have already used images such as the 'tree', 'bellows' and 'balloons'; this can be extended to the use of breathing body imagery. For example, during a foot or hand massage or reflexology session the patient can be invited to visualize breathing out and in through the webs of the fingers and toes, even choosing a colour(s) to imagine the flow of air and the benefits it brings, for example oxygen, freshness, a cooling breeze. We suggest splaying the fingers and toes on the in-breath and softening the hands/feet on the out-breath or using massage movements to the ends of the fingers/toes. (The combination of touch and imagery is explored in more detail in Chapter 12 on The HEARTS Process.) Patients can be invited to breathe in and out through the sides of the chest as though they have gills. This brings attention to the ribcage and shows how it can widen and then soften, pulling in and releasing the breath.

ENHANCING THE PHYSICAL ENVIRONMENT

The physical environment can be used to ease breathing; this can include mindful awareness of a hand-held or standing fan (Schwartzstein *et al.* 1987). Placing a bowl of ice between the fan and the patient can enhance the breeze. Exposing a limb can also bring attention to a 'feeling of the breeze on the skin'. Noticing actual or imagined windows, doors and even viewing pictures or videos of open spaces on mobile phones can augment a creative imagery journey. An example of using the physical environment, imagined or noticed, is described below.

Four-sided breathing (to calm and ease)

There are four-sided shapes wherever you look in a man-made environment. Some examples are doors, windows, mobile phones or even a page in this book.

Choose a vertical corner to begin. Start inhaling as you follow the arrow upwards to the next corner. Gently start exhaling as you follow along the horizontal line to the next corner of the shape.

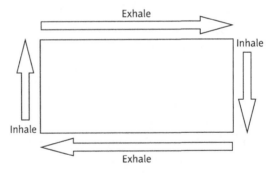

Figure 13.2: Four-sided breathing

Take a comfortable breath in as you journey downwards. Gently exhale along the next horizontal line to complete the shape. Repeat three times. (Figure 13.2 is suggested as a possible guide diagram for use with patients.)

A powerful variation is to allow the patient's attention to linger on the corners. Suggest that the patient really notices the space between the out-breath and the in-breath and how this can help him/

her to get a sense of an easy, rich breath. This will also help to regulate the carbon dioxide and oxygen levels in the blood.

This exercise can also be imagined. Patients can draw a shape in their mind's eye, and can close their eyes if it is more comfortable to do so. Many patients have told us that they imagine the shape to be a window or door that they can 'open' to let in a cool, moist breeze.

MINDFUL MOIST MOUTH (MMM)

Moistening the mouth can help make a dry throat, heat in the body and breathing feel more comfortable. Therapists typically offer patients water after a complementary therapy intervention, providing an opportunity to teach the MMM technique which combines mindfulness and imagery (Mackereth and Tomlinson 2014). First, suggest the patient swallows water normally, and notes where it touches the mouth and throat, and how far down the coolness tracks within the body. Second, invite the patient to hold and then consciously move water around the entire mouth before swallowing – repeat three times expanding on the awareness each time. Third, ask the patient to bring attention to how the mouth feels and where coolness has now tracked. Additionally, attention can be paid to the movement of the out-breath over a cooled tongue, so raising awareness of heat leaving the body. If the person is troubled by a dry throat or cough he/she can complete the process by sniffing and huffing and then swallowing on a comfortable and now moist mouth. A dry mouth can be a symptom of anxiety and distress, so bringing attention to MMM signals a change in the physical state that is associated with calmness and comfort.

STRAW BREATHING

Practising techniques that build respiratory capacity can be an ideal opportunity to introduce straw breathing. Ideally, this can be carried out when the person is at rest and without any immediate exertion.

For past or current smokers who want to change, this links to the hand-to-mouth association of drawing on a cigarette. Using a straw that has been cut to the length of a cigarette, invite the person to hold it as if smoking, but drawing in clear, fresh air. The empty tube encourages a 'focused pulling' in extending the in-breath. The patient is then encouraged to breathe out through the tube, which extends the out-breath; both these processes bring attention to accessory muscles during the respiratory cycle. The technique can be stacked with the aforementioned packing and emptying technique, so supporting and developing the use of the back muscles and belly in breathing.

THE STRETCH-YAWNING SYNDROME OR PANDICULATION – THE STRETCH, BREATHE AND YAWN TECHNIQUE

The 'stretch-yawning syndrome' (SYS) or pandiculation (stretching and yawning on waking) has been associated with the ability to reset the nervous system in animals, preparing them to respond to stressful situations (Bertolucci 2011). An exercise combining breathing, stretching and yawning, based on mimicking pandiculation, was developed to assist with calm diaphragmatic breathing (Mackereth 2012). The technique requires a 'stretchy man' or an elastic band (see Figures 13.3–13.6). We use a smiley, stretchy toy man, to remind patients (and carers) to breathe more efficiently by expanding the chest using the diaphragm (the large muscle at the base of the chest). With permission, the therapist rests his/her hands on the patient's lower back. The purpose is to raise awareness that these areas can be expanded, both outwards and downwards.

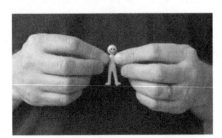

Figure 13.3: The stretchy man

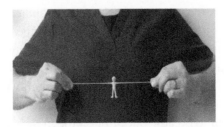

Figure 13.4: Expanding the chest and stretching the arms

Suggested instructions a therapist may give a patient

First: Stretch the arms of the man outwards as you take a comfortable breath in, and as you do so you will naturally expand your chest and naturally stretch the arms of the stretchy man. Then breathe out at your own pace as the yellow stretchy man's arms return to their normal size. This process is repeated a further three times (see Figure 13.4).

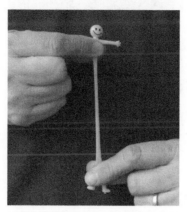

Figure 13.5: Stretching downwards by holding the shoulders and pulling down from the waist

Second: Hold the shoulders of the stretchy man and then pull the body down from the yellow stretchy man's waist as you take a slow breath in; repeat this process a further three times (see Figure 13.5).

Third: Take your attention to the stretchy man's legs. Stretch each leg in turn for two stretches, with four stretches done in total. As you do this, breathe comfortably into the tummy. Breathe out as the stretchy man's leg returns to its normal size. During this part of the technique you can stretch out your own legs in turn and then allow them to relax as you breathe out (see Figure 13.6).

Finally: We encourage you to yawn at the end of this technique. You may remember your therapist saying: 'You might find this technique triggers a yawn, if this happens [yawning] and it often does, just go with it, as it helps release tension from your body and makes breathing easier.'

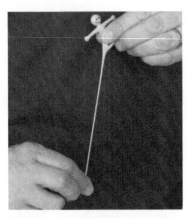

Figure 13.6: Pulling the legs downwards holding the waist

We recommend you practise the technique twice a day or more often as needed.

DO NOT FORGET THE THERAPIST'S OWN 'BREATH CUES'

Being aware of our own breathing and associated behaviours can be both useful in history taking, assessment, teaching and in our own self-care. Being mindful of our own breath cues can create opportunities for reflection, learning and change (Hunter 1993). Below are various statements, explored by therapists in relationship to the verbal and non-verbal communications and cues with patients, carers and colleagues. Some of the issues can trigger an intervention, for example asking about smoking and referring on with the encouragement that going smoke-free will help with improving respiratory function. Yawning and sniffing can be discussed as positive functions linked to breathing and the aforementioned techniques – pandiculation and sniffing and huffing.

Some therapists use attention to breathing to signal the beginning or end of a treatment; these breathing rituals have a place, but they need to be explained to patients and built on. For patients experiencing breathlessness, anxiety may be created, particularly if requested to 'breathe deeply', which may not be possible for them. Using invitational language and modelling the technique(s) can assist with patient understanding, literally giving permission to breath more easily within their whole body. Breathing in new ways can connect patients with themselves and others, releasing tension and energy so building new resilience (see Table 13.1).

Table 13.1: Breath cues – verbal and non-verbal communications

Breath cues	Possible interpretation
Taking a deep breath, holding it, tightening around the mouth…emitting a sigh/clicking	May signal contempt, frustration or disapproval
Short sharp breath and hold	Shock, disgust, don't want to take in
Sniffing, sneezing, coughing and gulping	May trigger worry, infection concern, curiosity or even anger; can be linked to fear and anxiety
Yawning	Boredom, fatigue, need to move on, breathe better
Smells – for example, tobacco, alcohol	Poor coping strategies – cannot take care/ notice self

ACUPRESSURE – COULD THIS THERAPY BE PART OF YOUR TOOLBOX?

Not all therapists are trained in acupuncture, but many may have an awareness of acupressure points. It is recommended that readers of this book pursue additional training in this area. By way of an introduction, we have identified a series of acupressure points that patients have found useful in managing cancer-related symptoms and concerns, such as breathing, cough and fatigue (Filshie *et al.* 1996; Molassiotis, Sylt and Diggins 2007). We suggest that therapists with little or no knowledge of acupressure could undertake a journey of investigation of this intervention; at the end you can decide to include the approach, to postpone it with plans for further training, or even reject the approach as part of your toolbox. As a therapist, you can decide on which techniques you feel comfortable with in terms of boundaries, accountability and responsibility for your work.

Key elements of using acupressure points are described here:

- Engagement – demonstrate the location of the points supported by laminated pictures and/or by recording on the patient's (or carer's) mobile telephone.

- Options/choices – always teach at least three points, so providing a choice based on ease of access, building comfort and preference for situations.

- Locus of control – it is important to acknowledge that rejecting an acupressure point is as important as choosing a preferred point. We would encourage patients to try out and test a combination of stackable resources.

- Future pacing – having tested and selected a 'package' of acupoints and other resources, patients can rehearse and plan their use of techniques in future situations.

Acupressure involves gentle pressure, which can be rhythmic, alternating or constant; the pressure is applied to a specific located point(s) for up to one minute. Typically, we suggest working the point two to three times per day either planned or when needed, for example prior to an activity, procedure or event or during an exacerbation of a symptom.

Theoretically there are differing views of the mechanism of action when using acupressure. These include the release of endorphins, stimulating the flow of chi (which is based on the meridian theory of traditional Chinese medicine) or expectations of the approach and placebo effects (Molassiotis *et al.* 2007; Vickers *et al.* 2005).

For those who are familiar with acupuncture and acupressure, useful points include the Conception Vessel 20 and 21, Lung 7 and Lung 9.

SUMMARY

In this chapter we have shared teachable techniques that patients, carers and even therapists can experience, review and test. They can be used either singularly or in combinations, depending on the patient's preference. The purpose of learning and practising these techniques is to help patients feel confident in using them prior to or during exertion, or when experiencing a challenging procedure. For therapists, these techniques can be applied to a variety of issues and concerns that go beyond breathlessness. They can be used where there is anxiety and distress related to other symptoms and living with cancer, its treatments and side-effects. Choice is the key to the potency of the resources; rejection of one or more of the techniques offered reinforces the value of the interventions chosen. Through incorporation of these techniques in our everyday practice, we, as breathing therapists, can support patients to breathe and live more calmly and comfortably.

REFERENCES

Bertolucci, L.F. (2011) 'Pandiculation: nature's way of maintaining the functional integrity of the myofascial system.' *Journal of Bodywork and Movement Therapies 15*, 3, 268–280.

Booth, S., Silvester, S., Todd, C. (2003) 'Breathlessness in cancer and chronic obstructive pulmonary disease: using a qualitative approach to describe the experience of patients and carers.' *Palliative and Supportive Care 1*, 4, 337–344.

Eriksen, M., Mackay, J., Ross, H. (2012) *The Tobacco Atlas* (4th edition, first edition date not available). Atlanta: American Cancer Society.

Filshie, J., Penn, K., Ashley, S., Davies, C.L. (1996) 'Acupuncture for the relief of cancer-related breathlessness.' *Palliative Medicine 10*, 145–150.

Hunter, V. (1993) 'Clinical cues in the breathing behaviors of patient and therapist.' *Clinical Social Work Journal 21*, 2, 161–178.

Hutson, M. and Ellis, R. (2006) (eds) *Textbook of Musculoskeletal Medicine*. Oxford: Oxford University Press.

Mackereth, P. (2012) 'Pandiculation: releasing anxiety during procedures.' *Anxiety Times* 83:14.

Mackereth, P. and Tomlinson, L. (2014) 'Procedure-related anxiety and needle phobia: rapid techniques to calm.' *Nursing in Practice 80*, 55–57.

Molassiotis, A., Sylt, P., Diggins, H. (2007) 'Complementary therapy medicine.' *Complementary Therapies in Medicine 15*, 4, 228–237.

Molassiotis, A., Lowe, M., Blackhall, F., Lorigan, P. (2010) 'A qualitative exploration of a respiratory distress symptom cluster in lung cancer: cough, breathlessness and fatigue.' *Lung Cancer 7*, 94–102.

Neuenschwander, H., Molto, A., Bianchi, M. (2006) 'External nasal dilator strips (ENDS) may improve breathlessness in cancer patients.' *Supportive Care in Cancer 14*, 4, 386–388.

Parkin, D.M., Boyd, L., Walker, L.C. (2011) 'The fraction of cancer attributable to lifestyle and environmental factors in the UK in 2010.' *British Journal of Cancer 105* Suppl: S77–81.

Ramponi, S. D. (2012) *Yoga & Breathing for Pregnancy & Birth*. Edinburgh: Purna.

Schwartzstein, R.M., Lahive, K., Pope, A., Weinberger, S.E., Weiss, J.W. (1987) 'Cold facial stimulation reduces breathlessness induced in normal subjects.' *American Review of Respiratory Disease 136*, 58–61.

Secretan, B., Straif, K., Baan, R., Grosse, Y. *et al.* (2009) 'A review of human carcinogens – Part E: tobacco, areca nut, alcohol smoke, and salted fish.' *The Lancet Oncology 10*, 11, 1033–1034.

Tishelman C., Petersson, L.M., Degner, L.F., Sprangers, M.A. (2007) 'Symptom prevalence, intensity, and distress in patients with inoperable lung cancer in relation to time of death.' *Journal of Clinical Oncology 25*, 5381–5389.

Vickers, A.J., Feinstein, M.B., Deng, G.E., Cassileth, B.R. (2005) 'Acupuncture for dyspnea in advanced cancer.' *British Medical Council Palliative Care 4:5* DOI:10.1186/1472-684X-4-5

Chapter 14

CARING FOR CARERS

Gwynneth Campbell and Rebecca Knowles

KEY WORDS

carer, chair massage, stress, anxiety, vigil, grief, CARER model

INTRODUCTION

This chapter focuses on how complementary therapies, particularly chair massage, can impact positively on the lives of informal caregivers of people with cancer. Examples of published research studies (2008–14) that outline the benefits of complementary therapies for carers are included. The challenges and concerns of carers are acknowledged and case studies are used to demonstrate ways in which chair massage has been beneficial in a hospital setting. Attention is drawn to the need for the therapist to be mindful of his/her posture while giving the treatment from a self-care perspective. The chapter concludes with an outline of the CARER model which summarizes the principles of working with carers.

OVERVIEW OF THE CHALLENGES OF CARERS

The diagnosis and process of cancer, or any life-threatening illness, is not only extremely stressful for patients, *but also* for their families, friends and work colleagues (Faulkner, Maguire and Regnard 1994; Mackereth, Campbell and Orrett 2012). People who are close to the patient embark on the journey as companions, witnessing investigations, waiting for diagnoses and observing the effects of the disease and treatment. Carers have an important role to play in the patient's cancer 'journey'. Physically, they accompany the patient to appointments and visit him/her in hospital; additionally, they accompany the patient mentally. This is often highlighted by the use of 'we' when describing the patient's treatment or appointments, as though they are going through it all with the patient (Mackereth *et al.* 2014).

Carers look to the future, hoping for a cure, yet preparing themselves for the possibility of loss. For the patient, there can be periods of relapse and remission bringing with them a readjustment of hopes and fears. Practical concerns can include loss of income if either the patient or carer has to stop working. Carers literally place their own lives on hold, and care for themselves often takes second place. Sometimes, normal activities such as hair washing or cooking a proper meal are overlooked; carers tell us they do not want to lose a precious moment away from their loved one. They may well have other family members, such as children, to care for, so they find themselves juggling their time and energy between home and hospital. Carers sometimes keep a bedside vigil in a hospital or hospice, sleeping fitfully on foldaway beds or chairs, adding to their physical and psychological stress. Higgins, Minter and Tarling (2011) have stated that the needs of carers are often overlooked by themselves and others around them; it is in the best interests of all concerned to offer carers support, comfort and tools for self-help and resilience.

Anxiety, fatigue, a sense of helplessness, being overwhelmed and pulled in different directions are all big stress factors. Complementary therapies have been shown to reduce stress and lower blood pressure and anxiety. Additionally, for carers, receiving a complementary therapy can provide a time to focus on themselves (Rexilius *et al.* 2002). Reviews of recently published research into the beneficial effects of complementary therapies for carers are shown in Table 14.1.

Table 14.1: Caring for carers research (2008–14)

Study	Objective	Design	Outcome measures	Results	Comments
Mackereth et al. (2008)	To gather patient and carer evaluations of a 20-minute chair massage treatment provided one afternoon a week in an outpatient waiting area.	Information gathered over a year included documented evaluation of chair massage, pre- and post-treatment wellbeing scores. Patients (n=224), carers (n=185).	Visual Analogue Scale (VAS)	Both patients and carers positively evaluated the treatment. Key benefits reported included relaxation, comfort, time out, treat, distraction and relief of anxiety. There were significant changes in self-reported wellbeing scores (p=<0.001), but no significant changes between scores for males and females.	This was an uncontrolled service evaluation utilizing subjective feedback and a VAS only.
Mackereth et al. (2014)	To assess the value of carers receiving complementary therapies to manage anxiety and stress related to witnessing their loved ones undergoing medical procedures.	Semi-structured interviews were conducted with carers and HADS scores were collected pre- and post-interview (n=10).	Hospital Anxiety and Depression Scale (HADS)	Post-interview HADS scores were reduced in all but one carer. Themes included being a carer faced with competing demands and limited resources, and being a witness and experiencing distress alongside their loved one.	All carers were appreciative of the complementary therapy support for loved ones and themselves. Some carers struggled to accept support and prioritize their own needs.

Nightingale and Stringer (2013)	To evaluate a Carers Complementary Therapy Project on a haematology and transplant unit.	Fifteen-minute chair massages were given to carers of the inpatients. Quantitative and qualitative data was collected on consultation forms and from questionnaires for a study period of 24 months (n=227).	Pre- and post-therapy scores.	138 carers presented with stress, 115 with sleep disturbance, 92 with worry and 88 with anxiety. The average pre-therapy 'feel good' score was 5/10 and the average post-therapy 'feel good' score was 8/10.	The data suggests that the Carers Project facilitated positive change in the physical, mental and emotional state of carers.
Curry, Donaghy and Hughes (2008)	To determine if it would be feasible to conduct a randomized controlled trial on the effectiveness of aromatherapy on carers of patients with cancer.	Pilot randomized controlled trial in a local outpatient clinic. Participants were randomly allocated to receive six sessions of either aromatherapy massage or relaxation (n=10).	Hospital Anxiety and Depression Scale. Measure Your Medical Outcome Profile. Taken pre- and post-intervention and follow-up.	There were clinically significant improvements following aromatherapy massage for anxiety, depression and sleep. No changes were observed following relaxation.	The results suggest that aromatherapy massage may be of benefit for people caring for patients with advanced cancer, in alleviating anxiety and depression. The information provided enabled the design of a full randomized controlled trial.

cont.

Study	Objective	Design	Outcome measures	Results	Comments
Higgins, Minter and Tarling (2011)	To provide good quality support to informal, unpaid carers of patients using the inpatient unit at Hartlepool and District Hospice.	The therapies offered were aromatherapy, reflexology, reiki, Indian head massage and foot massage. The complementary therapist provided the service either at the hospice or in the carer's home. Each carer received four treatments, one for an hour each week (n=15).	An evaluation form was provided following each treatment.	All carers rated their treatment as 'excellent', with 100% commenting that they felt 'more relaxed'. Carers also reported additional benefits including reduced anxiety, lowering of stress levels and an improved sense of wellbeing. No carers reported 'no noticeable benefit'.	The offer of complementary therapies in their own home was enthusiastically received. The treatments allowed carers to feel comfortable and valued, with an increased sense of resilience. Spending quality time with the therapist gave an opportunity to raise concerns which could then be passed on to an appropriate professional.
Cronfalk, Strang and Ternestedt (2009)	To explore relatives' experiences of receiving soft tissue massage as a support supplement while caring for a dying family member at home.	Relatives received soft tissue massage (hand or foot) nine times (25 minutes) in their homes. Open-ended semi-structured tape-recorded interviews were conducted once per relative after the nine sessions of massage, using qualitative content analysis (n=19).	Interviews (qualitative data).	Soft tissue massage gave the relatives feelings of 'being cared for', 'body vitality' and 'peace of mind'. For a while, they put worries of daily life aside as they just experienced 'being'. During massage, it became apparent that body and mind are constituted of an indestructible completeness. The overarching theme was 'inner power, physical strength and existential wellbeing in their daily lives'.	All relatives experienced soft tissue massage positively. It could be an option to comfort and support relatives in palliative home care.

Research studies have indicated that therapies other than massage can also benefit carers in their time of need, including yoga, mindfulness and art therapy (Baines 2011; Farquhar *et al.* 2014; Fish *et al.* 2014; Lang and Lim 2014; McDonald, Burjan and Martin 2006).

Chair massage for carers in hospital settings

The therapeutic use of massage in different forms has been recognized for thousands of years in many cultures around the world. One particular form of massage, namely chair massage, has become popular in recent years with a huge rise of 'on-site' massage in workplaces and healthcare settings. In the 1980s, David Palmer, an experienced massage instructor, developed this form of seated massage, using an ergonomically designed and portable, padded, foldable chair (Palmer 1998). The design of the chair fully supports the whole body and provides an opportunity for short, seated, fully clothed treatments that can be given anywhere, so enabling opportunities for immediate relaxation (see Figure 14.1).

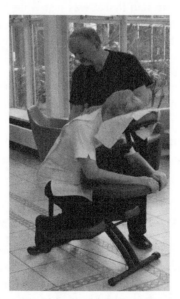

Figure 14.1: A massage chair supporting the whole body

The style of massage that Palmer developed was focused on acupressure and meridian theory. However, muscle-based techniques are also advocated by chair massage instructors when incorporating adaptations for the individual recipient and also to prevent injury to practitioners (Baines 2011; Greene 1995; Mackereth and Campbell 2002; Pyves and Woodhouse 2003). Gentle stroking and holding can be a very helpful style of massage to use for a stressed carer (see Case study 14.1).

Case study 14.1: A short, soothing treatment for a stressed carer

Janelle's husband was very ill in hospital. She had been recommended to attend the drop-in complementary therapy service by nurses on the ward. Janelle was very stressed with juggling family responsibilities and visits to the hospital. On arrival at the drop-in, she appeared very agitated, talking and breathing quickly; she said she only wanted to be away from her husband for a short time.

A ten-minute chair massage was agreed, and after an initial consultation Janelle was settled into the chair. The therapist used gentle effleurage and reassuring holding, slowing the strokes down as the massage progressed. When Janelle sat up, she said that it was just what she had needed; she especially liked the light stroking, and had found that comforting. Her breathing was noticeably slower, and she looked and sounded much calmer.

Chair massage can be a way to safely receive massage when privacy is not available and removal of clothing is impractical. The portability of the chair enables therapists to deliver the treatment to carers wherever they are in the hospital, whether that is in a dayroom, a drop-in relaxation session, in the garden or simply by the bedside (see Case study 14.2).

Case study 14.2: Supporting a 'vigil'

A patient's partner, Jack, had been sleeping with considerable discomfort in a chair beside the patient's bed for two weeks. He reported feeling tense and exhausted, but was afraid to leave his partner in case her condition deteriorated. Following a referral made by a member of staff, he received a chair massage in the patient's room. Jack reported relaxing completely during the treatment and muscle tension easing. After resting for a few moments, he returned to his vigil, noticeably refreshed, and lay down on the bed, snuggling into his partner.

In addition to healthcare staff initiating referrals, a therapist may identify a need and offer a chair massage to relatives. Case study 14.3 highlights how the chair and its 'embracing' shape can provide a discreet 'cocoon' for receiving empathic touch and, potentially, releasing tears privately (Mackereth *et al.* 2012).

Case study 14.3: Release of emotional tension

Rose had been maintaining a vigil at her husband's bedside. The therapist first provided a gentle foot massage for her partner and then offered chair massage to Rose. When Rose realized she could have the treatment by his bedside, she agreed. Rose reported being very anxious and had not slept for the last two days. After the treatment she appeared less tense and began to cry. She said, 'The massage really touched me and I just couldn't hold back the tears any longer.'

We have observed that when a carer shifts from an anxious place, through receiving massage, a relaxation response may be triggered in the patient's body (Mackereth *et al.* 2012). Case study 14.4 illustrates this phenomenon of 'body empathy', a two-way connection between people who care about each other (Shaw 2003).

Case study 14.4: A two-way connection between carer and patient

Lucy was sitting with her dying mother, Beth, in her hospital room, both appearing anxious and scared. Lucy reported that seeing her mother with a breathing mask and drains and tubes was alarming, and she was finding it hard to see her mother beneath it all.

After giving a foot massage to Beth, the therapist offered Lucy a chair massage. Despite Beth saying, 'Lucy, please have a massage,' Lucy said she did not want to move away from her bedside. The therapist suggested that she could have a head and shoulder massage without oil, so Lucy could continue to hold Beth's hand. Lucy agreed and afterwards looked more relaxed. Beth gripped Lucy's hand and smiled and closed her eyes looking more content.

Daniels (2003) believes that carers should be encouraged to seek out and request the kind of support they need to maintain their role.

When clothed chair massage is offered in a waiting area, or an open ward, carers are able to see the treatment in 'real time'. Relatives or close friends often accompany a patient to outpatient appointments and being able to see the treatment, and being aware of its availability, can encourage them to request a session for themselves (see Case study 14.5).

Case study 14.5: Chair massage in a waiting area

Chair massage was being offered to both patients and carers in a busy waiting area. After watching people coming off the chair looking more relaxed, and realizing this service was on offer, Martha, whose sister was waiting to see the consultant, requested a treatment for herself. After the treatment she reported that her headache had gone and she felt less anxious and more able to be fully present for her sister.

PRACTICAL CONSIDERATIONS AND ADAPTATIONS

Being comfortable throughout the treatment is important and the recipient is encouraged to indicate any discomfort, or desire to stop the treatment at any time. Ongoing monitoring is crucial and the therapist needs to notice, for example, if the recipient becomes fidgety or if there are any changes in breathing patterns. It is also important to monitor how comfortable you are as a therapist. Pyves and Mackereth (2002) argue that we need to be mindful of our posture and balance to protect our bodies from unnecessary strain and damage. Ways of working without undue strain are shown in Figures 14.2 and 14.3. Notice the use of soft forearms in both photographs. This increases the contact area and provides a cocoon of holding, stroking and gentle 'leaning in' without exerting pressure.

For people using a wheelchair, the 'half chair' can be used. This is a headrest on an adjustable support which can be secured on to a table or massage couch, enabling a wheelchair to be drawn close to the half chair.

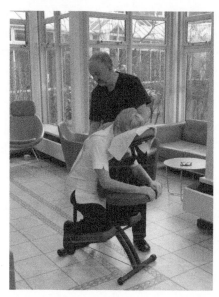

Figure 14.2: Sitting on a chair or a stool behind the receiver to avoid unnecessary strain on the back

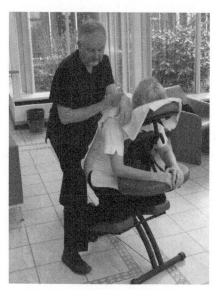

Figure 14.3: Notice the soft use of forearms to save unnecessary strain on the hands

CHECKING FOR CONTRAINDICATIONS

The therapist always needs to check contraindications to massage, and assess whether the carer can sit comfortably and feel 'embraced' by the chair, before agreeing on the content and style of massage. Examples of contraindications include:

- unable to mount chair

- unable to consent, for example the individual is confused and disorientated, has taken sedatives or narcotics, or excess alcohol

- recent surgery or injury

- raised temperature or feeling dizzy or unwell

- unstable blood pressure or heart problems

- extreme or unexplained pain.

TEACHING CARERS

Partners or friends may like to learn a skill that offers something positive they can do for a loved one. Experiencing and/or delivering a hand or foot massage can be beneficial for both receiver and giver (Cullen *et al.* 2000). In our experience, carers have asked to learn some massage techniques that they can do when the therapist is not available. We suggest that the carer first observes the therapist providing a hand or foot massage. The carer can then be invited to join the therapist in a massage, mirroring the movements on the other hand or foot. Two powerful experiences of teaching massage to carers are illustrated in Case study 14.6.

Case study 14.6: Acceptance and feeling valued

Denis was visiting his partner John. Denis confided in the ward's massage therapist that he was worried about showing affection to John by holding his hand in front of other visitors and patients. The therapist suggested teaching Denis hand massage as a practical way of relaxing and comforting John. Denis watched as the therapist demonstrated some hand massage techniques on one of John's hands, then he joined in, working on the opposite hand and mirroring the techniques.

After watching for a while, the son of a patient in the opposite bed asked the therapist to teach him to massage his father's feet. While the son was learning the foot massage his dad closed his eyes and then said a few minutes later, 'Hey, I can't tell the difference between who is doing which foot...you've got a new career son.'

During her next visit to the ward, the therapist noticed Denis chatting to other visitors, holding his partner's hand.

THE CARER MODEL

We have developed a simple model (the CARER model) to encapsulate the principles and approaches explored in this chapter. *Comfort* includes explaining to carers how complementary therapies, and in particular massage, can give physical and emotional support at a time when they may need it most. Prior to any intervention, the therapist can *Assess* a carer's health needs and wellbeing using a simple consultation document, ideally alongside an evaluation tool. A particularly useful approach is for the carer to give a pre- and post-treatment score on a 0 to 10 Visual Analogue Scale. An example is the Feeling Good Thermometer (Field 2000). The therapist can suggest or provide *Resources*, which may include self-help tools, such as an aromastick, relaxation and breathing techniques (see Chapters 8, 10 and 13). Details of local organizations where complementary therapies and other sources of advice can also be a useful resource. Learning self-care and simple techniques to use with their family can be *Empowering* and help build *Resilience* to sustain them at the present time and in the future.

A summary of the CARER model

- Comfort and a complementary therapy intervention.

- Assess wellbeing and health needs of carers.

- Resources and referrals for carers considered.

- Empowering carers through teaching and learning self-care and interventions.

- Resilience: a combination of elements to build and sustain carers during and beyond caring for someone with cancer.

SUMMARY

The massage chair has been found to be a most valuable and flexible resource enabling the therapist to work in a variety of ways and situations where access to a complementary therapy treatment would not have been possible. This chapter has described some of the potential benefits of chair massage in supporting carers through some of the difficult and stressful times of living with someone with cancer. These difficulties have been acknowledged and the benefits of chair massage have been described using case studies as illustrations as to how chair massage has been used to good effect. Additionally, attention has been drawn to the need for therapists to be mindful of their own posture and safety issues when doing treatments, as well as those of the individual with whom they are working.

REFERENCES

Baines, E. (2011) 'Evaluating an adapted mindfulness meditation course for use in palliative care setting.' *British Medical Journal Supportive and Palliative Care 1*, 2, 267–268.

Cronfalk, B.S., Strang, P., Ternestedt, B.M. (2009) 'Inner power, physical strength and existential well-being in daily life: relatives' experiences of receiving soft tissue massage in palliative home care.' *Journal of Clinical Nursing 18*, 15, 2225–2233.

Cullen, C., Field, T., Escalona, A., Hartshorn, K. (2000) 'Father-infant interactions are enhanced by massage therapy.' *Early Child Development and Care 164*, 10, 41–47.

Curry, S., Donaghy, K., Hughes, C. (2008) 'The effectiveness of aromatherapy massage of improving psychosocial well-being of carers of patients with advanced progressive cancer: a pilot randomized controlled clinical trial.' *International Journal of Clinical Aromatherapy 5*, 2, 9–16.

Daniels, R. (2003) *The Carer's Guide In Cancer Lifeline Kit.* Bristol: Health Creation.

Faulkner, A., Maguire, P. and Regnard, C. (1994) 'Breaking bad news: a flow diagram.' *Palliative Medicine, 8*, 2, 145–151.

Farquhar, M.C., Prevost, A.T., McCrone, P., Brafman-Price, B. *et al.* (2014) 'Is a specialist breathlessness service more effective and cost-effective for patients with advanced cancer and their carers than standard care? Findings of a mixed-method randomized controlled trial.' *BMC Medicine 12*, 1, 194.

Faulkner, A., Maguire, P. and Regnard, C. (1994) 'Breaking bad news: a flow diagram.' *Palliative Medicine, 8*, 2, 145–151.

Field, T. (2000) *Touch Therapy.* London: Churchill Livingstone.

Fish, J.A., Ettridge, K., Sharplin, G.R., Hancock, B., Knott, V.E. (2014) 'Mindfulness-based cancer stress management: impact of a mindfulness-based program on psychological distress and quality of life.' *European Journal of Cancer Care 23*, 3, 413–421.

Greene, L. (1995) *Save Your Hands.* Florida: Gilded Age Press.

Higgins, S., Minter, H., Tarling, C. (2011) 'Complementary therapies for carers: a pilot study.' *European Journal of Palliative Care 18*, 6, 285–287.

Lang, D. and Lim, L. (2014) 'Effects of art therapy for family caregivers of cancer patients: a systematic review.' *JBI Database of Systematic Reviews and Implementation Reports 12,* 4, 374–394.

Mackereth, P., Mehrez, A.J., Hackman, E., Knowles, R. (2014) 'The value of complementary therapies for carers witnessing patients' medical procedures.' *Cancer Nursing Practice 13,* 9, 32–38.

Mackereth, P., Campbell, G., Maycock, P., Hennings, J. *et al.* (2008) 'Chair massage for patients and carers: a pilot service in an outpatient setting of a cancer care hospital.' *Complementary Therapies in Clinical Practice 14,* 2, 136–142.

Mackereth, P., Campbell, G., Orrett, L. (2012) 'Private moment in a public space: massage for distressed carers.' *Biodynamic Massage 15,* 1, 4–7.

Mackereth, P. and Campbell, G. (2002) 'Chair massage: attention and touch in 15 minutes.' *Palliative and Cancer Matters Newsletter No. 25,* 2–6.

McDonald, A., Burjan, E., Martin, S. (2006) 'Yoga for patients and carers in a palliative day care setting.' *International Journal of Palliative Nursing 12,* 1, 519–523.

Nightingale, L. and Stringer, J. (2013) 'Complementary therapy for carers on a transplant unit.' *Complementary Therapies in Clinical Practice 19,* 3, 119–127.

Palmer, D. (1998) 'Therapeutic chair massage.' *Positive Health, 32.* Available at www. positivehealth.com/article/massage/a-brief-history-of-chair-massage, accessed on 29 November 2015.

Pyves, G. and Mackereth, P. A. (2002) 'Practising Safely and Effectively: Introducing the 'No Hands' Approach, A Paradigm Shift in the Theory and Practice of Reflexology.' In: P. Mackereth and D. Tiran (eds) *Clinical Reflexology: A Guide for Health Professionals.* London: Churchill Livingstone.

Pyves, G. and Woodhouse. D. (eds) (2003) *NO HANDS Chair Massage.* Halifax: Shizen Publications.

Rexilius, S. Mundt, A. Megel, M. *et al.* (2002) 'Therapeutic effects of massage therapy and healing touch on caregivers of patients undergoing autologous hematopoietic stem cell transplant.' *Oncology Nursing Forum 29,* 3, 35–44.

Shaw, R. (2003) *The Embodied Psychotherapist: The Therapist's Body Story.* Hove, East Sussex: Brunner-Routledge.

Chapter 15

SPIRITUALITY AND WORKING ETHICALLY AT THE END OF LIFE

Dr Peter A. Mackereth and Reverend Kevin Dunn

KEY WORDS
religion, spirituality, ritual, purpose, touch, end of life

INTRODUCTION

Offering complementary therapies to patients (and their carers) when time is limited can present complex challenges. This chapter explores the role of ritual and spirituality and religion at the end of life. Rather than prescribe the role of the therapist, the authors raise issues for reflection. First, the Reverend Kevin Dunn explores the concept of ritual as it relates to spirituality and religion and possible considerations for end-of-life care. Second, Dr Peter A. Mackereth reflects on these concepts, utilizing end-of-life case studies and ethical and professional considerations in practice. In reading this chapter, please consider these questions linked to end-of-life care that have arisen in training with therapists:

- What happens if the person dies while I am in the room?

- What if some family or staff do not want me to offer interventions or support at this time?

- Should I ask carers at the bedside if they would like a treatment?

- What is my purpose in being there?

- What do I do if the patient becomes unconscious during the treatment?

- What if families ask me to attend the funeral?

(based on Mackereth and Sexton 2016)

RITUAL AND SPIRITUALITY

In palliative and end-of-life care, the role of spirituality, as distinct from religion, has been the subject of considerable attention, since the beginning of the modern hospice movement, yet definitions of what spirituality is remain elusive. Murray and Zentner (1989) define spirituality as, 'A quality that goes beyond religious affiliation, that strives for inspirations, reverence, awe, meaning and purpose, even in those who do not believe in any god. The spiritual dimension tries to be in harmony with the universe, strives for answers about the infinite, and comes into focus when the person faces emotional stress, physical illness or death' (p.259). However, in *The Dying Soul*, Cobb (2001) comments that, 'Spiritual for some is a vacuous word because it is so bland or unfathomable, made more elusive by being considered sacrosanct' (p.13). In spite of the ongoing difficulty in pinning down a range of things that 'spirituality' might mean, there seems to be a broad consensus on some of its common features. It is, for example, related to religion; Walter (2002) suggests that spirituality is adopted 'by those who wish to move beyond, or distance themselves from, institutional religion' (p.6). In the context of palliative care, Cobb (2001) suggests that spirituality deals with whatever is 'of ultimate reality and worth for a person' and relates to matters of 'fundamental importance' (p.13). A person's spirituality is closely linked to, and, in part is the expression of, their deepest held and most precious beliefs about their world.

Ritual may be defined as 'a religious or solemn ceremony involving a series of actions performed in a prescribed order' (Concise Oxford English Dictionary 2006). Walter (1994) comments that rituals may evolve out of more personal and individual needs, rather than those of traditional religion. However, there are some clearly identified rituals depending on the culture and religion of an individual – these include behaviours surrounding births, christenings, weddings, deaths and funerals. Ritual, whether religious or not, permeates human life, from the ritual greeting of a seemingly casual handshake to the complex civic rituals of national and political life. What is perhaps most significant in end-of-life care is to recognize what ritual can achieve, and to utilize it where it can be of benefit. A common feature of ritual is that the process denotes activity that is more *symbolic* (a representation) than *instrumental* (achieving an aim); the activity is not undertaken primarily to achieve a concrete purpose. Nevertheless, the boundaries may be blurred. The activity of eating with a purpose to overcome hunger may sometimes be inseparable from all the symbolic activities of the communal sharing of food. There are many possible ways of describing the benefits of ritual to human life, but Driver (1998) usefully divides these benefits under the headings of order, community and transformation.

ORDER

The element of order comes about through rituals being essentially repetitive and rhythmic. Today's ritual will be more or less the same as yesterday's ritual, and it will be more or less the same tomorrow. Speaking of Christian ritual, Kavanagh (1982) says, '[R]hythm, which organizes repetition, makes things memorable, as in music, poetry, rhetoric, architecture... It fuses people to their values and forges them to a common purpose' (p.28).

COMMUNITY

In spiritual care, people in crisis often ask to be reminded of prayers, ritual or scriptural texts, or religious music learned long ago, often in childhood. These ritual repetitions are able to bear a great weight of memory and association and can vividly evoke happier and more peaceful times. Sometimes the associations that these texts carry count for more than the meanings of the texts themselves; it may not be wise for a carer to subject the texts to too much analysis or critique. In Jewish and Christian traditions, an example is the use of psalm texts, some of which can shock modern sensibilities by their frank portrayal of negative feelings, but which nevertheless remain a source of comfort to those familiar with them.

Much ritual, especially perhaps in the more formal religious setting, is communal in nature, for example, the Christian Mass and the Jummah prayers of Islam. However, this is not an accidental feature of ritual: ritual does not only happen in community, it can assert and form community. One of the outcomes of this aspect of ritual is to 'visibly to restore the harmonious relationships' between individuals and with their social environment (Helman 2007, p.240).

People nearing the end of their lives often express the need to restore broken relationships, and the use of ritual to facilitate this is another important aspect of spiritual care. This process often involves the interplay of some very sensitive and sometimes negative emotions. Ritual, by its imposition of order, can channel these emotions in relatively safe ways to achieve restoration and reconciliation. Driver (1998) observes that, 'Ritual controls emotion while releasing it, and guides it while letting it run. Even in a time of grief, ritual lets joy be present through the permission to cry, lets tears become laughter, if they will...all this in the presence of communal assertiveness' (p.156).

TRANSFORMATION

Possibly the most powerful use of ritual in end-of-life care is in the area of transformation or transition. The term 'rite of passage' is commonly used in everyday speech, but in its technical, anthropological usage, the term refers to a specific kind of ritual, or set of rituals, evolved or designed to manage transition between different stages of life – childhood and adulthood, singleness and marriage, life and death. Post-death rituals that help the bereaved re-assimilate into their society can also often be described as rites of passage (see Case study 15.1).

Case study 15.1: An example of a post-death ritual

In life, David, a therapist with the complementary therapy team, had been a guitarist and a singer and he loved to dance. It was a shock to everyone when he died suddenly and his lively personality was missed by everyone. He was always ready to assist at events with his singing and playing the guitar and had helped to organize a memorial events for a therapist who died two years previously.

David died following a very short illness – his patients were told as David had been running a number of clinics and group sessions. The team organized a celebration evening, with the hospital's chaplain, whom David knew well. Patients attended, along with colleagues and family. Rather than sit quietly at the back of the room, the group of patients stood up (holding hands) and in turn spoke about their memories and connections with David. At the end of the evening David's favourite piece of 'fun' music was played and everyone in the room stood up spontaneously and danced and hugged each other.

RITES OF PASSAGE

Rites of passage are characterized by three phases. These are described differently by different writers, but Arnold van Gennep, who first studied rites of passage in traditional cultures, used the terms 'separation', 'transition' and 'incorporation' (Bowie 2000, pp.162–163). The person undergoing the rite of passage passes through each stage accompanied by rituals of various kinds, and, especially in the middle stage, is often helped by a spiritual guide or mentor. Bowie (2000) describes a familiar rite of passage as a traditional western pattern of the transition from being single to being married. When a couple planned to marry there were various rituals of *separation* from their former families, culminating in the wedding ceremony. (The 'giving away' of a bride by her father remained an eloquent rite of separation, even when it no longer had any social or economic meaning.) The *transition* was the honeymoon, which traditionally followed the communal meal after the wedding. The couple who, in a sense, still weren't quite married, went away by themselves for a period of time. It was only when they were incorporated into their social circle after the honeymoon that they were regarded as a fully married couple; the incorporation stereotypically involved rites, such as the woman being carried over the threshold of their new home. A full account of the role of rites of passage cannot be given here, but it is easy to see how the pattern of these rites can be applied to the person nearing the end of their life. If the person is dying in hospital, there seems to be an instinct among professional carers to grant them seclusion, and as much spiritual and emotional guidance as they need during the time of transition. During this time, appropriate spiritual care can give reassurance and comfort, help with the expression of emotion, and facilitate desired reconciliations. The final 'incorporation' here, of course, is death itself. In turn, death marks the beginning of a new set of rites of passage for the bereaved as they transition to a new life, without the person who was once perhaps central to their lives.

THE PLACE OF THERAPIES IN END-OF-LIFE CARE

Receiving complementary therapies at end of life can be welcomed, questioned or even given little thought. As part of an end-of-life ritual, the family may exclude non-essential staff from coming into the 'dying room', the motive often being to create a protected and secluded family space for transition and privacy. Clinical staff may also hold similar views about the need for privacy, and may question whether there is a place for complementary therapists at this time. One concession may be to enlist therapists to help in supporting members of the family. The ritual of the bedside vigil can be exhausting and stressful for family and friends (see Figure 15.1), yet there is often a reluctance to leave the loved one for fear that they will be needed or the person may pass away in their absence (see Chapter 14). Health professionals, themselves, may seek out complementary therapies to help them cope, or avoid the burnout of working in cancer care (Wilson *et al.* 2007).

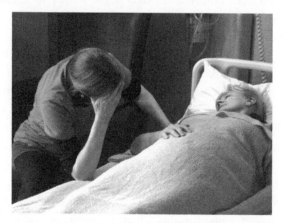

Figure 15.1: The vigil by the bedside

A team of complementary therapists who offer massage and other interventions in hospital and hospice settings is a relatively new phenomenon and may be outside the experience of many patients and their carers. Physiologically, the dying person may start to 'shut down', with circulation compromised and limbs cold to touch. Using approaches which make use of other sensory experiences such as aromas, guided imagery or HEARTS may be helpful, even when a person is close to death. The gentle repetitive, soothing and rhythmic movements of a simple hand massage, as well as focused holding of the body, can create a protective cocoon, connecting people and spaces (Garnett 2003).

CONSENT, ENGAGEMENT AND 'GOOD ENOUGH' ENDINGS

Obtaining consent can be a ritual in itself. We cannot always predict a repeatable and consistent outcome for massage, a HEARTS treatment or guided imagery. Gentle touch and holding can be an expression of caring from the therapist's view; however, the recipient's experience may not accord with this intention. Past experience of abusive touch and/or association with medical procedures may trigger a very different physical and emotional response in the recipient, or even in witnesses (family and friends), who may have their own experiences of touch and their responses to it. As therapists, the challenge in attending to the dying and their family and carers is the ability to sensitively and non-intrusively evaluate our work.

Patients may be in a state of altered consciousness (see Case study 15.2) and it may not always be appropriate (or possible) to gather direct feedback at this time. It is essential that therapists monitor non-verbal communications, picking up cues that might indicate the relaxation response in both patients and carers. Interviews with therapists suggest that providing complementary therapy to carers in close proximity to the patient can result in the patient also becoming calmer (Mehrez *et al.* 2015). Overhearing interactions with carers and therapists about receiving a massage could, in part, explain this response. It may be that a carer's own non-verbal communication indicates his/her calmer state. Changes, such as sighing, slowing breathing and a noticeable softness in the voice may comfort a patient who is concerned about their carer's own wellbeing.

Case study 15.2: In and out of consciousness

Aashi had been receiving complementary therapy as an outpatient prior to admission; she knew she might experience some loss of consciousness during the period of palliative brain radiotherapy sessions. Therapists provided daily sessions of foot and hand massage by agreement, even when Aashi appeared very drowsy. Each time, explanations were given and non-verbal cues observed. Four days post-radiotherapy, Aashi regained full consciousness and reported how wonderful it was to have received massage during her stay, even remembering the names of the massage therapists. She said the ritual of a daily massage helped her to feel cared for, connected and less fearful of the treatment.

When entering a room where therapies are being provided, health professionals (and visitors) will often make positive comments about what they see, or, if essential oils have been provided, the smell in the room. Terms like 'haven' and 'sanctuary' have been used; one visitor commented, 'It feels like the walls have been massaged too.'

Making use of memory and patterns of behaviour can create a shift in state for both the patient and those who are present. Some may be in constant vigil, others may be making a brief, and possibly a last, visit to a loved one (see Case study 15.3).

Case study 15.3: Around the kitchen table

Emily had requested a head massage; all her family (five adults) were in the room and appeared tense and subdued. The therapist suggested to Emily, 'I can combine this with some visualization...how about sitting around your lovely big pine kitchen table?' (On a previous visit, Emily had shared how her kitchen was the heart of her home, with the 'kettle always on'.) Emily smiled and nodded. The therapist invited her family to remember a time after a wedding, a party, any celebration or any other event when everyone piled into the kitchen for 'a cuppa' and a slice of one of Emily's sumptuous cakes. All closed their eyes spontaneously and settled back in their chairs. After the ten minutes of visualization the therapist gently bought them back into the room. Conversations flowed about 'being around the kitchen table'; there was laughter, with incidents and conversations remembered and recounted. Emily even managed a giggle and closed her eyes smiling. She died in her sleep during the night with the family present.

BEING NON-CLINICAL

A challenge for therapists is being aware as to how they present at the bedside. In hospitals, the wearing of uniforms is linked to notions of a professional appearance, coupled with infection control concerns and safety issues. Uniforms can be both protective and offer a boundary, physically and psychologically. For some patients, seeing someone in a uniform may provide reassurance and may help in recognition of someone in a defined role and a position (Spragley and Francis 2006). Infection control has seen the demise of the tie and long sleeves and the emphasis is on proper hand hygiene and appropriate use of protective gloves. MacDonald (2014) argues that there is case for 'always' wearing gloves for massage in a clinical setting with concern for skin contamination from possible infection and drug metabolites, for example from chemotherapy. In reviewing the available literature, there is no evidence that levels of metabolites on the skin pose a problem for massage therapists (see Figure 15.2).

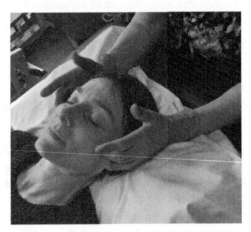

Figure 15.2: Massage with gloves. What do you think?

Importantly, adhering to hand-washing procedures should be adequate in preventing cross-contamination. Gloves need only be worn when a therapist has cuts, abrasions or dermatitis, or where the patient is being barrier nursed, or has a known skin condition, such as impetigo (Mackereth and Ferguson 2015). Tony Nicklinson, a patient, was interviewed by a journalist about the experience of 24-hour care as he approached the end of his life. Tony expressed distress that he was only touched through protective gloves, saying, 'Carers would pet my dog, but they wouldn't touch me without gloves' (Nazarko 2011).

MY PURPOSE IN BEING THERE

If a complementary therapist has been a regular feature in the patient's journey, it is likely that the family will want the treatments to continue in the patient's last weeks and days, particularly if it brings comfort and relaxation. Importantly, carers often ask the therapist to teach them simple massage techniques, so that they can provide these when the therapist is not on site. It is possible for two therapists to attend patients at end of life, with the second therapist offering treatments to carers in the room, or to provide paired working. It is important to think about our purpose in being there at this time – it has to be about providing support and comfort, not attempting to sort out family disputes or providing religious guidance. It is not unusual for patients (and carers) to experience an existential shift, questioning their own lives and beliefs, relationships difficulties, past mistakes, and wasted opportunities. Equally, there can be an acceptance and an appreciation of a life lived and the love received. As therapists, we can listen and witness with touch and other techniques, facilitating and communicating comfort, care and respect with our presence and intention to help.

ADAPTING AND REMAINING IN CONNECTION

For some patients at end of life, the ability to maintain contact with the therapist can be a challenge, due to either the dying process or fatigue. Interventions needs to be individualized and caution should be exercised not to overtax the patient; 15–20-minute treatments (or less), with some time to rest quietly, may be much appreciated by patients (and carers). The quality of treatment and the sensitivity of the touch are more important than the duration and areas of the body to be treated (Mackereth and Maycock 2012).

Patients may drift in and out of consciousness; if you are there for any length of time the patient may have forgotten you were there and could be startled to see you. Importantly, circulation may be reduced and while gentle massage and reflexology may help to warm the feet, it may be a better option to work with the hands, as these are more accessible and within vision. This is particularly important as most patients at end of life will be lying on their side supported by cushions, rather than sitting in an upright position. Working with the patient's hands can also provide opportunities for carers to observe the techniques and mirror work on the other hand. Remember, carers may have spent hours at the hospice, hospital or in the patient's home and may not had a wash or change of clothes for days (see Chapter 14), so if you are offering foot massage or reflexology, always arrive equipped with wipes and fresh towels.

Touch and presence can often sustain a connection, so it is unlikely that a patient will die during an intervention; indeed, the most common time period for dying is in the early hours of the morning. Every moment of being with, and every act of love provided, will be stored in a carer's mind. 'A good death' is always the goal and can be a profound experience for future situations and for when we finally reach this point in our own lives. Meetings between family members at funerals and future end-of-life situations will inevitably recall past experiences, such as, 'Do you remember how relaxed mum was after her head and hands massage? She had a lovely smile on her face.'

THE WOUNDED AND HEALING SELF

It is an honour and a privilege to be invited into an intimate space to provide therapies at end of life; however, it is very important to look after yourself as well as carrying out your duties as a therapist. Working in an acute cancer care setting or a hospice over time can sometimes feel like 'serial bereavement'. Being part of a supportive wider multidisciplinary team can help to sustain resilience. Regular clinical supervision sessions, always respecting confidentiality, can provide a space to reflect on the experience of being with someone who is dying (or has died) (Mackereth and Mehrez 2012). Dying is a time of transition – the experience for those at the bedside will remain memorable, precious and can inform future dying experiences. Current guidelines for care of the dying place the patient and carer at the heart of what we do as health professionals. The emphasis is that the care should be provided with compassion, respect and sensitivity (National Council for Palliative Care 2013). A helpful online resource for families (and therapists), entitled 'What to expect when someone important to you is dying: A guide for carers, families and friends of dying people', is also available (National Council for Palliative Care 2015).

If you have come to know a patient over a period of time or the experience has been intense, the family may ask you to attend the person's funeral or memorial event. Such an invitation is an honour, but attendance is always voluntary. Always discuss the invitation with your manager and should you wish to attend, consider going with another member of the team involved in the patient's care for support.

Remembering and celebrating the person who has passed can be an important transition; it can also be an emotional experience for all those who have been touched by that person.

It is important for therapists to question and reflect on why they are drawn to working in healthcare and, in particular, hospice settings. When recruiting therapists it is useful to ask, 'What motivates you to want to work here?' and 'What past experiences, views and understanding do you have of cancer and caring for people who are dying?' The concept of the 'wounded healer' tells us much about the beliefs and expectations of health professionals and therapists. Here, the concept is linked to the ancient Greek myth of the Centaur, Chiron, who developed his compassion, skill and empathy as a healer from living with his own wound (Cawthorn 2006).

SUMMARY

Aside from ensuring that you are competent to practise safely, obtaining informed consent and ensuring comfort at all times are essential tenets when providing complementary therapy interventions to patients (and carers). Below are practice issues for reflection:

- Recognize your limitations and seek skills in adapting treatments to ensure safety and comfort at end of life.

- Offer and ensure consent for short and gentle sessions for patients – the treatment may include noticing physical cues, for example, if the patient sighs and relaxes, or if they become restless and/or withdraw a limb.

- Inform, involve and provide interventions for carers, such as teaching self-help techniques or offering to provide a short hand or foot treatment.

- Remember that for some patients, and even for carers, this might be a time of withdrawal and the family gathering around the person – always respect the wishes of family and patients for privacy.

- Remember that families may share their feelings and past experiences, and there may even be anger and unresolved issues – it is important to listen, be non-judgemental and avoid giving advice or guidance (religious or otherwise).

- Engage with the Chaplaincy Team (and the wider multidisciplinary team) to ensure seamless and appropriate support, such as spiritual care, pain relief and review of other symptoms.

REFERENCES

Bowie, F. (2000) *The Anthropology of Religion.* Oxford: Blackwell.

Cobb, M. (2001) *The Dying Soul: Spiritual Care at the End of Life.* London: Open University Press.

Concise Oxford English Dictionary (2006) Oxford: Oxford University Press.

Cawthorn, A. (2006) 'Working with the Denied Body.' In P. Mackereth, and A. Carter (eds) *Massage and Bodywork: Adapting Therapies for Cancer Care.* London: Elsevier.

Driver, T.F. (1998) *Liberating Rites.* Boulder, CO: Westview Press.

Garnett, M. (2003) 'Sustaining the cocoon: the emotional inoculation produced by complementary therapies in palliative care.' *European Journal of Cancer Care. 12,* 129–136.

Helman, C.G. (2007) *Culture, Health and Illness.* (5th edition) London: Hodder Arnold.

Kavanagh, A. (1982) *Elements of Rite.* Collegeville: Pueblo.

MacDonald, G. (2014) *Medicine Hands* (3rd edition) Scotland: Findhorn Press.

Mackereth, P. and Ferguson, A. (2015) 'Gloves off.' *International Therapist 113,* 22–24.

Mackereth, P. and Sexton, J. (2016) 'End of life and reflexology: creating a loving cocoon.' *Reflexions, March Edition* 13–14.

Mackereth, P. and Mehrez, A. (2012) 'Super-vision: helping to develop and support your practice.' *International Therapist 99,* 30–32.

Mackereth, P. and Maycock P. (2012) 'Reflexology in palliative and supportive care: the case model.' *Reflexions, June Edition,* 16–18.

Mehrez, A., Knowles, R., Mackereth, P., Hackman, E. (2015) 'The value of stress relieving techniques.' *Cancer Nursing Practice 14,* 4, 14–21.

Murray, R. B. and Zentner, J.B. (1989) *Nursing Concepts for Health Promotion.* London: Prentice-Hall.

National Council for Palliative Care (2013) 'The end of life care strategy: new ambitions. 'Available at www.ncpc.org.uk/sites/default/files/End%20of%20Life%20Care%20Strategy%20New%20Ambitions%20Report_WEB.pdf, accessed on 14 January 2016.

National Council for Palliative Care (2015) *'What to expect when someone important to you is dying: a guide for carers, families and friends of dying people.'* Available at www.ncpc.org.uk/sites/default/files/user/documents/What_to_Expect_FINAL_WEB.pdf, accessed on 14 January 2016.

Nazarko L (2011) 'Carers would pet my dog but they wouldn't touch me without gloves.' *Nursing Times 107,* 2, 14.

Spragley, F. and Francis, K. (2006) 'Nursing uniforms: professional symbol or outdated relic?' *Nursing Management 37,* 10, 55–58.

Walter, T. (1994) *The Revival of Death.* Abingdon: Routledge.

Walter, T. (2002) 'Spirituality in palliative care: opportunity or burden?' *Palliative Medicine 16,* 2, 133–139.

Wilson, K., Ganley, A., Mackereth, P., Roswell, V. (2007) 'Subsidized complementary therapies for staff and volunteers at a regional cancer centre a formative study.' *European Journal of Cancer Care 16,* 291–299.

LIST OF EDITORS

Ann Carter BA, Dip Health Ed, Cert Ed, Cert NLP has a background in training and health promotion; she has worked as a complementary therapist and teacher since 1989 in both hospices and in the acute sector. From 2000 to 2008, Ann co-ordinated the complementary therapy service across the three sites of a large hospice in Manchester. She also helped establish the Christie CALM service and facilitated Relaxation Classes at its main hospital site. From 2008, Ann became education co-lead for the Christie Complementary Therapies Training Programme and was responsible for innovating the Diploma in Complementary Therapies in Cancer Care and a management course for co-ordinators. To meet the needs of individuals at different stages of illness, Ann developed The HEARTS Process and has delivered many workshops to therapists and healthcare professionals throughout the UK and Ireland. In addition to her training role, Ann has been a regular speaker at conferences in the UK, and has also contributed to conferences in Dublin, Tokyo and Toronto. She has also contributed numerous articles and chapters to complementary therapy journals.

Dr Peter A. Mackereth PhD, MA Dip (N) London, RNT, RGN is a registered nurse, and has worked in intensive care, neurology and oncology. He has also worked as a nurse lecturer and reader within the university setting. Peter has an MA in medical ethics and has completed a PhD project examining reflexology versus relaxation training for people living with multiple sclerosis. He has trained in acupuncture, hypnotherapy, body psychotherapy, massage and reflexology. For the last 15 years Peter has worked as clinical lead for a complementary health and wellbeing service at The Christie, an acute oncology cancer centre. He has authored a number of papers, chapters and books and speaks nationally and internationally on complementary therapies, cancer care and smoking cessation. Recent and ongoing studies include assisting with needle anxiety and phobia, fatigue, peripheral neuropathy and insomnia.

LIST OF CONTRIBUTORS

Gwynneth Campbell BA (Hons), PGCE completed her first training in massage in 1983 and works as a complementary therapist in private practice and at The Christie, Manchester. She has taught complementary therapies in various settings for many years, and teaches on the Adapting Massage for Cancer Care programme, including chair and head massage. Her wide-ranging massage skills have been influenced by several modalities, including NO HANDS® Massage, reflexology, shiatsu and subtle healing techniques. She is also a practitioner and teacher of Chiron Healing® and a committee member of the International Association of Chiron Healers Inc.

Graeme Donald PhD, BSc, DPSN, RN, Dip Hypno is a lecturer in adult nursing at the University of Manchester. His therapy practices include acupuncture, hypnotherapy and delivering mindfulness meditation sessions. He has clinical experience in medical assessment and oncology and has researched a variety of complementary therapies in clinical practice while previously working as a nurse researcher and therapist at The Christie. His interests include person-centred care, complementary medicine and stress management, considered in his doctoral thesis evaluating mindfulness meditation in the stress management of people living with HIV.

Reverend Kevin Dunn BSc, MA was recently a chaplaincy and humanities manager at The Christie, Manchester. After a first degree in physics, he was a junior research assistant in the Department of Meteorology. He was ordained as an Anglican priest in 1993 and has been involved in healthcare chaplaincy since 1995. He has particular interests in literature, the arts and spirituality, and in the philosophy of healthcare.

Timothy Jackson MSc, SRN, SCM, RNSM, Onc Cert has over 40 years' NHS and voluntary sector experience, and 30 years' working in cancer care, including specialist palliative care as a clinician, manager and director in the London area. His track record includes working operationally and strategically across complex organizational boundaries, including managed care networks and nationally. Tim has worked as a nurse/management consultant for cancer service reviews and redesign. He is also advisor to the Supreme Council of Health for the introduction of a quality assurance framework for state and private care providers within Qatar.

Rebecca Knowles BSc (Hons) completed a number of training courses in areas such as cancer datasets and critical appraisal during the time she worked as a clinical research assistant at The Christie. Currently, she has had three journal articles published, two in *Cancer Nursing Practice* and one in *Wounds UK*. Prior to this she was awarded a first class honours degree in food and nutrition from Manchester Metropolitan University. She completed a gap-year placement working as an assistant nutritionist for Manchester City Council and went on to work as a clinical trials assistant for Intertek Clinical Research Services.

Paula Maycock LI Biol, Dip Hypno, LIAcu, MIFPA, MAR is a clinical hypnotherapist with a focus on health, wellbeing and managing stress. A senior therapist within The Christie, as well as working in private practice, Paula places emphasis on supporting patients and carers through their experiences using an integrated therapy approach. This incorporates a range of therapies and amalgamates qualifications in clinical aromatherapy, reflexology and acupuncture with biochemistry and microbiology along with many years experience of working with people living with long-term illness. Paula is also proactive in promoting and supporting the use of complementary therapies and hypnotherapy in the successful attainment of a smoke-free lifestyle. Paula has published and lectured within medical research and complementary medicine research fields.

Anita Mehrez RGN, Postgraduate Dip Psycho-Oncology, Dip Hypno trained as a nurse and worked in haematology, oncology, neurology and neurosurgery. She began her training in complementary therapies in 1997. Anita worked for several years at St Ann's Hospice, providing aromatherapy massage alongside a physiotherapist in a symptom control clinic for women following treatment for breast cancer. She is deputy clinical lead in complementary therapies at The Christie, where she uses an integrated approach incorporating aromatherapy, clinical hypnotherapy, acupuncture, massage and reflexology. She is also a master in the NO HANDS® Massage method. Anita has co-authored a number of papers and book chapters and presents regularly at conferences and workshops.

Lydia Nightingale BA (Hons), C&G 7407, Dip Hypno, Dip Complementary Therapies in Cancer Care is a specialist palliative care complementary therapist at The Christie and also has her own private practice. She has experience in cancer care, hospice care, HIV, community and outreach settings. At The Christie, she works within the multidisciplinary Supportive and Palliative Care Team and co-ordinates the provision of complementary therapists for palliative and end-of-life inpatients and their carers. She provides massage, HEARTS, guided imagery, relaxation and hypnotherapy. Lydia was lead author for a service evaluation paper 'Complementary therapy for carers on a transplant unit', published in the journal, *Complementary Therapies in Clinical Practice*.

Dr Jacqui Stringer PhD, BSc, RGN, TIDHA, MIFPA, Winston Churchill Fellow 2003 is co-lead for the complementary therapy team and lead for tissue viability at The Christie. Her focus is on the clinical management of patients with complex physiological and psychological needs, with a specific interest in working with patients who have haematological conditions. The role includes maintaining a clinical caseload where standard licensed medications are used in conjunction with off-licence essential oil preparations to facilitate maximum healing and symptom support, for example in wound care. The role involves research, education and product development relating to her clinical work.

Lynne Tomlinson BSc Hons, D.Hyp BSCH (Assoc), MBACP Counselling, Post-Grad Dip Cognitive Behavioural Psycho-therapy integrates clinical hypnotherapy, mindfulness practice and complementary therapies with cognitive behavioural protocols and counselling models. Lynne works as a senior clinical hypnotherapist with the Christie Head and Neck Project and the HypnoCalm Pre-operative Care Project. Lynne specializes in providing emergency interventions to enable patients to work through the challenges of treatment. She is the senior tutor for the Integrative Hypnotherapy Diploma Course at The Christie and has developed bespoke courses for midwives and counsellors and yoga for birth instructors. Lynne provides supervision for hypnotherapists and is currently studying for a Master's in cognitive behaviour psychotherapy.

SUBJECT INDEX

Sub-headings in *italics* indicate tables and boxes.

AUTHOR INDEX